EMQs and MCQs for the FRCOphth Part 2

D1471688

Patrick Chiam MBBCh(Hons) FRCOphth MBA

Ophthalmic Registrar

Eye Unit

Stoke Mandeville Hospital

Aylesbury

Buckinghamshire

United Kingdom

To my family

Front cover: Toxoplasma retinochoroiditis

Contents

Preface...iv

Breakdown of previous FRCOphth written exam questions by topic
- EMQ..v
- MCQ...vi

EMQ Paper 1...1

EMQ Paper 1 Answers...24

MCQ Paper 1...36

MCQ Paper 1 Answers..53

EMQ Paper 2...62

EMQ Paper 2 Answers..86

MCQ Paper 2...100

MCQ Paper 2 Answers..117

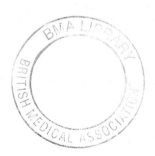

Preface

The FRCOphth Part 2 exam was introduced in September 2008. Thus far, with the exception of the first diet, each exam result has been analysed and published on the Royal College of Ophthalmologists website (www.rcophth.co.uk). The median pass rate for the written part (so far) is about 50% and only successful candidates are allowed to proceed to the clinical part. To date there has not been any books or many online questions available to give candidates a flavour of the exam.

In this book, I have written the EMQs and MCQs based on the latest FRCOphth Part 2 exam format and syllabus. The papers reflect the style of the exam. There is a significant amount of basic science and research/statistics questions. I have included a table of question breakdown by topic from the past papers. Each of the EMQ and MCQ papers in this book is written based on similar question spread.

The majority of the EMQs stems consist of 10 options. There are 45 stems and 2 questions per stem. Occasionally, only 8 or 9 options are available and this is stated at the beginning of the question. The time allowed is 3 hours. Most of the questions are in clinical scenario forms. The MCQ paper consists of choosing the best answer out of four options. There are 90 questions and the duration of the exam is 2 hours. Questions on disease inheritance, health economics, refraction, optics and esoteric conditions have been asked in the past EMQ and MCQ papers. The highest numbers of questions have been on therapeutics and ophthalmic investigations.

Candidates are advised to be familiar with the Royal College of Ophthalmologists and the National Institute for Health and Clinical Excellence guidelines. The General Medical Council guidance on various topics such as good medical practice, confidentially, etc should be revised. The outcome of landmark studies in glaucoma, age related macular degeneration, retinal vein occlusion, diabetic retinopathy should form part of the exam revision.

This book is written with the intention to provide candidates the likely nature and scope of the questions encountered in the exam. I have included many similar questions that were used in the previous exam papers. For candidates who already feel well prepared, the EMQ and MCQ papers can be attempted as a mock exam. All the best!

Patrick Chiam

EMQ	Sep-08	Feb-09	Sep-09	Feb-10	Sep-10	Feb-11	Paper 1	Paper 2
Uveitis	4	4	4	2	2	6	4	4
Paediatrics	4	2	4	6	4	4	4	6
Vitreoretinal	4	4	2	0	2	6	2	4
Medical retina	8	10	14	12	8	8	12	10
Strabismus	6	4	4	4	4	4	4	4
Oculoplastics and orbit	4	4	8	2	4	4	6	5
Cornea/external eye	4	7	6	6	6	7	6	6
Trauma	2	2	2	4	2	4	2	2
Cataract/lens	2	4	2	4	4	4	4	4
Glaucoma	6	4	6	4	4	4	4	6
Oncology				2			0	1
Neurology	12	13	12	12	12	10	12	12
Medicine	10	4	2	2	4	2	2	2
Pathology/genetics	4	6	8	4	6	4	8	6
Optics/refraction	0	2	2	2	2	2	2	2
Anatomy/physiology					2	0		
Pharmacology	8	8	8	12	12	11	10	8
Ophthalmic and neuroimaging	6	6	0	6	12	4	4	4
Statistics and epidemiology	4	2	0	4		4	2	2
Research	2	4	6	2	2		2	2
Total	90	90	90	90	90	88*	90	90

*2 questions excluded from the exam

MCQ	Sep-08	Feb-09	Sep-09	Feb-10	Sep-10	Feb-11	Paper 1	Paper 2
Anatomy & embryology	2	3	3	2	2	4	2	3
Microbiology	3	4	4	4	3	3	4	3
Optics	6	2	5	2	7	2	4	4
Genetics	3	2	3	1	1	2	2	2
Pathology	8	6	4	6	6	5	6	6
Physiology	2	0	0	3	3	0	2	2
Cataract	1	3	3	3	2	3	3	2
Neurology & pupils	8	3	5	4	5	4	5	5
Glaucoma	2	2	2	2	3	3	3	3
Strabismus	2	5	2	2	3	3	3	3
Paediatrics	1	3	4	3	2	2	3	2
Vitreoretinal	2	4	2	3	2	4	3	4
Medical retina & uveitis	6	6	4	6	5	4	6	5
Oculoplastics and orbit	2	1	3	2	2	3	3	3
Cornea	3	3	2	3	4	4	3	4
Oncology					1	2		2
Pharmacology & therapeutics	7	12	10	8	9	8	8	9
Ophthalmic & neuroimaging	14	14	16	20	13	17	16	14
Orthoptics	3	3	4					
Statistics and research	7	4	5	5	8	7	5	7
Medicolegal	3	3	1	4	2	1	2	1
Health economics	1	1	1	1	1	1	1	1
Ethics	1	0	0	2	1	2	1	1
General medicine	1	3	2	2	1	1	2	1
Guidelines	2	3	5	2	3	4	3	3
Total	90	90	90	90	89	89	90	90

EMQ Paper 1

A) Juvenile retinoschisis
B) Lowe syndrome
C) Blue-cone monochromatism
D) Leber congenital amaurosis
E) CSNB with myopia (Schubert-Bornschein)
F) Leber optic neuropathy
G) Kearn-Sayre syndrome
H) Alport syndrome
I) Gyrate atrophy
J) Sorsby retinopathy

Select the most likely condition for the statements below.

1) This condition is inherited as X-linked dominant.

2) This is an autosomal dominant disorder.

A) Sarcoidosis
B) Behcet disease
C) Vogt-Koyanagi-Harada syndrome
D) Polyarteritis nodosa
E) Thyroidopathy
F) Wegener granulomatosis
G) Systemic lupus erythematosus
H) Tuberculosis
I) Syphilis
J) Stevens-Johnson syndrome

Choose the most likely diagnosis for each situation.

3) This condition causes a net-like rash on the abdomen.

4) Pyoderma gangrenosum is a feature of this disorder.

A) Chloramphenicol
B) Tetracycline
C) Gentamicin
D) Cefradine
E) Fusidic acid
F) Trimethoprim
G) Vancomycin
H) Ofloxacin
I) Penicillin
J) Amoxicillin

Choose the appropriate antibiotic for each description.

5) Inhibits 50S subunit of ribosome, hindering bacterial protein synthesis.

6) Impedes DNA gyrase thereby inhibits DNA replication.

A) Preseptal cellulitis
B) Orbital cellulitis
C) Optic nerve glioma
D) Rhabdomyosarcoma
E) Thyroid orbitopathy
F) Diffuse choroidal haemangioma
G) Orbital myositis
H) Spheno-orbital encephalocele
I) Dacryoadenitis
J) Tolosa-Hunt syndrome

Select the most appropriate diagnosis for each presentation.

7) A 22-year-old patient presents to her GP with progressive visual loss in the both eyes. She has patches of brown macules on her torso and rubbery papules around her wrists. Her younger brother, mother and uncle have similar lesions.

8) A 17-year-old complains of diplopia with a painful, proptosed and closed left eye. There is lid oedema and chemosis. The white blood count is 6.5×10^9/litre and the temperature is 36.8^0C.

A) Cyclopentolate
B) Pilocarpine
C) Guanethidine
D) Acetylcholine
E) Atropine
F) Proxymethocaine
G) Phenylephrine
H) Tropicamide
I) Ecothiopate
J) Physostigmine

Select the likely drug for each description.

9) Acts on sympathetic and parasympathetic autonomic ganglia.

10) Reduces lid retraction caused by thyroid eye disease.

A) Aspergillosis
B) HIV microvasculopathy
C) Herpes simplex uveitis
D) CMV retinitis
E) Tuberculosis retinitis
F) Molluscum contagiosum
G) Kaposi sarcoma
H) Herpes simplex keratitis
I) Blepharitis
J) Sicca syndrome

For the following questions, select the most likely diagnosis.

11) An African teenager who has been incompliant with her antiretroviral treatment presents with painless, severe visual blurring in one eye. Her CD4+ count is 40cells/µl.

12) A 35-year-old stewardess has recently been diagnosed with HIV. He is not on any antiretroviral treatment and his CD4+ count is 800cells/µl. He complains of gritty red eyes.

A) Ciclosporin
B) Sirolimus
C) 5-fluorouracil
D) Tacrolimus
E) Methotrexate
F) Cyclophosphamide
G) Mycophenolate mofetil
H) Prednisolone
I) Azathioprine
J) Rituximab

Select the likely drug for the following questions.

13) Allopurinol enhances the effect this immunosuppressant.

14) Causes halitosis and gingival hyperplasia.

A) Infantile esotropia
B) Fully accommodative esotropia
C) Partially accommodative esotropia
D) Non-refractive convergence excess
E) Near esotropia
F) Simulated intermittent distance exotropia
G) True intermittent distance exotropia
H) Near exotropia
I) Secondary exotropia
J) Consecutive exotropia

Select the most likely condition for each clinical examination.

15) A toddler with intermittent squint noted by her parent. The visual acuities are 6/6 in both eyes. Alternate cover test shows distant exotropia with good recovery.

Prism cover test: +3.0D both eyes, 10PD BI for near, 40PD BI for distant

Refraction: RE +2.50/-0.50 X 180   LE +2.75/-0.50 X 165

16) A 4-year-old with a convergent squint. The visual acuity are 6/6 OD, 6/18 OS. Alternate cover test shows left esotropia with and without glasses for distant.

Prism cover test: without glasses 45PD BO; with glasses 25PD BO for distant

Refraction: RE +4.50DS   LE +6.00DS

A) Duane syndrome type 1
B) Duane syndrome type 2
C) Duane syndrome type 3
D) Duane syndrome type 4
E) Congential exotropia
F) Congenital fibrosis of the extraocular muscles
G) Mobius syndrome
H) Strabismus fixus
I) Brown syndrome
J) Double elevator palsy

Select the most appropriate diagnosis for each patient.

17) An infant with limited adduction of the left eye and normal abduction. There is a small degree of left exotropia and narrowing of the left palpebral fissure on dextroversion.

18) A 5-year-old with severe limitation of horizontal gaze. Both eyes are orthophoric in the primary position with normal down gaze. The Bell's phenomenon is present.

A) Pars plana vitrectomy and inferior sclera buckle
B) Drainage of subretinal fluid and inferior scleral buckle
C) Inferior cryotherapy and 360^0 scleral buckle
D) Drainage of subretinal fluid and inferior cryotherapy
E) Pars plana vitrectomy and silicone oil
F) Pars plana vitrectomy, ILM peel and fluid-air exchange
G) Pars plana vitrectomy, ILM peel and 12% of C_3F_8
H) Pars plana vitrectomy, ILM peel and 20% of SF_6
I) Pars plana vitrectomy, ILM peel and 40% of SF_6
J) Pars plana vitrectomy, ILM peel and silicone oil

Choose the most appropriate surgical repair method for the conditions mentioned.

19) A 25-year-old sustains a blunt trauma to the left eye 2 years ago. He complains that his left superior visual field has been progressively blurry over the past 3 months. The left visual acuity is 6/5 and there is a macular-on bullous inferior retinal dialysis.

20) A 75-year-old is keen to have a full thickness macular hole surgery repair, however, is unable to posture face down. She is pseudophakic.

A) Treat with prostaglandin analogue and review 1 to 4 months later
B) Treat with topical β-blocker and review 1 to 4 months later
C) Treat with topical α-agonist and review 1 to 4 months later
D) Treat with prostaglandin analogue and review 6 to 12 months later
E) Treat with topical β-blocker and review 6 to 12 months later
F) Perform 360^0 laser trabeculoplasty and review 1 to 4 months later
G) Perform 180^0 laser trabeculoplasty and review 1 to 4 months later
H) No treatment, and review in 2 to 4 months
I) No treatment, and review in 12 to 24 months
J) Discharge patient

According to the 2009 National Institute for Health and Clinical Excellence (NICE) guidelines, what is the recommended management for the ocular hypertensive patients below?

21) A 55-year-old healthy bus driver with a wide opened iridocorneal angle, cornea thickness of 570μm and IOP of 27mmHg.

22) A 75-year-old referred by her optometrist with an IOP of 23mmHg. Pachymetry reveals a cornea thickness of 535μm. There is no family history of glaucoma. She is only on ramipril for hypertension.

A) Best macular dystrophy
B) Familial dominant drusen
C) Stargardt disease
D) Fundus flavimaculatus
E) Central serous chorioretinopathy
F) Sjogren-Larsson syndrome
G) Tay-Sachs disease
H) Enhanced S-cone syndrome
I) Nougaret congenital nyctalopia
J) Oguchi disease

Choose the likely diagnosis for each patient.

23) A 16-year-old student struggles with her exam revision and complains of poor central vision to her optometrist. Her visual acuity with glasses is 6/24 bilaterally. The optometrist does not find any abnormally on dilated fundal examination.

24) A 12-year-old was noted to be accident prone in the dark on a camping trip. He occasionally complains of difficulty with his vision in bright light. The optometrist mentioned a peculiar pattern of pigmentation at the periphery of the retina.

A) Lattice dystrophy
B) Granular dystrophy
C) Macular dystrophy
D) Schnyder dystrophy
E) Labrador keratopathy
F) Hunter syndrome
G) Scheie syndrome
H) Sanfilippo syndrome
I) Morquio syndrome
J) Maroteaux-Lamy syndrome

Select the most appropriate condition for each description.

25) The underlying pathology is stained with Masson trichrome.

26) A 65-year-old has severe clouding of the cornea and pigmentary retinopathy. He has an IQ of 120.

There are only 9 options available for this question.

A) Asthma
B) Polyarteritis nodosa
C) Anaphylaxis
D) Wegener's granulomatosis
E) Penicillin allergy
F) Graves disease
G) Temporal arteritis
H) Systemic lupus erythematosus
I) Marginal keratitis

Choose the most appropriate condition for the type of hypersensitivity.

27) Type II

28) Type IV

A) -3.00 / -1.50 X 135
B) -1.00 / -2.50 X 45
C) -1.00 / -2.50 X 135
D) -3.00 / -4.50 X 135
E) -4.50 / +1.50 X 135
F) +0.50 / -2.00 X 90
G) +0.50 DS
H) -1.50 / +2.00 X 180
I) -1.50 / +2.00 X 90
J) + 0.50 DC X 180

Select the refraction outcome for each examination.

29) Retinoscopy with the beam vertically requires a +2.00D lens to neutralise the reflex at 2/3m. No lens is required to produce the same effect with horizontal beam retinoscopy.

30) An examiner at working distance of 1/2m obtained a neutral reflex with -1.00D lens at 135^0 meridian and -2.50D at 45^0.

A) Orbital cellulitis
B) Thrombophlebitis of the orbital vein
C) Direct carotid-cavernous fistula
D) Indirect carotid-cavernous fistula
E) Thyroid eye disease
F) Blow-out fracture of the orbital floor
G) Blow-out fracture of the medial orbital wall
H) Zygomatic wall fracture
I) Orbital roof fracture
J) 'Trapdoor' blow-out fracture of the orbital floor

Choose the most likely diagnosis for each patient.

31) A 33-year-old motorist had a road traffic accident two weeks ago. He presents with sudden onset of blurring, diplopia, chemosis and injected conjunctival in the left eye. He complains of an annoying whooshing sound in his head.

32) A 12-year-old boy fell on the handle of his bicycle. There is marked restriction and severe pain in the right eye in upgaze. He has been feeling nauseous and vomited twice already. There is mild lid oedema, but no haemorrhage or globe rupture. The nurse mentions his heart rate was 40beats/min.

A) Weber syndrome
B) Benedikt syndrome
C) Nothangel syndrome
D) Claude syndrome
E) Parinaud dorsal midbrain syndrome
F) Foville syndrome
G) Millard-Gubler syndrome
H) Raymond syndrome
I) Ramsay-Hunt syndrome
J) Mobius syndrome

Select the most like diagnosis for each patient.

33) A 74-year-old develops sudden onset diplopia. The medical registrar finds right intentional tremor and dysdiadochokinesis. The right pupil is dilated and the eye is limited in adduction, up- and down-gaze.

34) A 30-year-old gentleman complains of increasing right deafness. He has diplopia looking into the distance. He also has slight weakness and numbness on the right side of his face.

A) Topical prostaglandin analogue, steroid and atropine
B) PRP and topical prostaglandin analogue, steroid and atropine
C) PRP, intracameral bevacizumab and topical prostaglandin analogue
D) Ciliary body cyclodiode and topical anti-glaucoma, steroid and atropine
E) PRP, intracameral bevacizumab and ciliary body cyclodiode
F) Macular grid laser and repeat as necessary
G) Intravitreal bevacizumab and repeat as necessary
H) Intravitreal bevacizumab and macular grid laser
I) Intravitreal triamcinolone acetonide (Kenalog)
J) Topical steroid, and oral acetazolamide

According to the Royal College of Ophthalmologists recommendations for retinal vein occlusion management, choose the most appropriate treatment option for each patient.

35) A 70-year-old with 6 months history of central retinal vein occlusion develops florid rubeosis iridis in an opened iridocorneal angle. There is no macular oedema. The acuity is 6/60, and IOP 23mmHg.

36) A 68-year-old was diagnosed with non-ischaemic central retinal vein occlusion two months ago. The OCT scan reveals a central macular thickness of 400μm and visual acuity of 6/12.

A) Morgagnian cataract
B) Sun-flower cataract
C) Stellate posterior subcapsular cataract
D) Anterior capsular cataract
E) Radial cortical cataract
F) Cerulean (blue-dot) cataract
G) Oil droplet cataract
H) Membranous cataract
I) Lamellar cataract
J) Anterior polar cataract

Select the most likely type of cataract for each case.

37) A 25-year-old with progressive dementia, akinetic rigidity in his upper limbs and jaundice.

38) An infant fails to thrive and has been vomiting. He is found to have poor fundal red reflex. A reducing substance was found in the urine after milk feeding recently.

A) Gram negative bacillus
B) Gram negative diplococci
C) Gram negative spirochete
D) Gram negative rod
E) Gram negative coccobacilli
F) Gram positive cocci coagulase positive
G) Gram positive cocci coagulase negative
H) Gram positive cocci β-haemolytic
I) Gram positive cocci α-haemolytic
J) Gram positive cocci γ-haemolytic

Classify the bacteria accordingly.

39) Neisseria gonorrhoea

40) Staphylococcus epidermidis

A) Wilcoxon test
B) Mann-Whitney test
C) Paired *t* test
D) Unpaired *t* test
E) Friedman test
F) Kruskal-Wallis test
G) One-way analysis of variance
H) Spearman correlation
I) Pearson correlation
J) Multiple linear regression

Select the most appropriate statistical test for each study objective.

41) Comparing the IOP reduction in two groups of patient on different anti-glaucoma treatment.

42) The correlation between the numbers of ranibizumab injection with visual acuity at 12-month follow-up.

A) Bitemporal hemianopia with denser inferotemporal defect
B) Bitemporal hemianopia with denser superotemporal defect
C) Central bitemporal hemianopia
D) Binasal hemianopia
E) Left congruous homonymous hemianopia
F) Left inferior homonymous quadrantanopia
G) Left superior homonymous quadrantanopia
H) Right congruous homonymous hemianopia
I) Right inferior homonymous quadrantanopia
J) Right superior homonymous quadrantanopia

Select the most likely visual field defect for each case.

43) A 15-year-old boy who is very short for his age and obese frequently bumps into pedestrians on the street. The paediatricians are investigating him for delayed sexual maturation and frequent headache.

44) A right-handed patient finds it difficult to perform simple arithmetic and distinguish the fingers on his hand. He seems disorientated between his left and right limbs. He has asymmetrical optokinetic nystagmus.

A) CT
B) MRI T1 weighted with STIR
C) MRI T2 weighted with STIR
D) MRI T2 weighted with FLAIR
E) MR angiography
F) Skull X-ray
G) Contrast dacryocystography
H) CT dacryocystography
I) MR dacryocystography
J) Dacryoscintigraphy

Select the most appropriate imaging for each case.

45) A patient with recent exacerbation of thyroid eye disease.

46) A patient with epiphora who has patent syringing of the tear passage with minimal reflux on numerous occasion. Anterior segment examination is unremarkable.

A) Acute posterior multifocal placoid pigment epitheliopathy (APMPPE)
B) Serpiginous choroidopathy
C) Birdshot choroidopathy
D) Multiple evanescent white-dot syndrome
E) Punctuate inner choroidopathy (PIC)
F) Vogt-Koyanagi-Harada syndrome
G) Acute zonal occult outer retinopathy (AZOOR)
H) Progressive subretinal fibrosis and uveitis syndrome
I) Multifocal choroiditis with panuveitis (MCP)
J) Acute idiopathic blind spot enlargement syndrome (AIBSES)

Choose the probable diagnosis for each patient.

47) A 27-year-old gentleman who has just recovered from a flu-like illness, complained of visual impairment in the left eye. Examination reveals mild vitritis, multiple deep creamy flat plaques scattered in the posterior pole and adjacent the superior and inferior arcades.

48) A 30-year-old lady presents with photopsia and occasional blurred vision. The visual field test shows multiple areas of reduced sensitivity. Her visual acuities are 6/5. Dilated fundoscopy and fluorescein angiography are unremarkable. The ERG reveals delayed implicit time of the 30Hz cone flicker response. EOG shows a reduction of the light rise.

A) ANCHOR
B) EXCITE
C) FOCUS
D) MARINA
E) PIER
F) PrONTO
G) SAILOR
H) SUSTAIN
I) VIP
J) VISION

Select the appropriate trial which corresponds with each statement.

49) Monthly loading dose of ranibizumab for 3 months followed by treatment on an as-required-basis if the visual acuity is reduced by 5 letters on the LogMAR chart or the OCT showed thickening of the retina by 100μm.

50) A third of eyes with minimally classic or occult choroidal neovascularisation experienced a visual acuity gain of ≥ 15 letters from baseline to 12 months.

A) Lateral tarsal strip
B) Lateral tarsal strip and Quickert suture
C) Wies procedure
D) Jones procedure
E) Lower lid wedge resection
F) Tarsal fracture
G) Medial canthoplasty
H) Medial canthal resection
I) Medial tarso-conjunctival diamond excision and lateral tarsal strip
J) Kuhnt-Symanowski procedure

Select the most appropriate procedure for each condition.

51) This patient has significant horizontal lower lid laxity, minimal vertical laxity and entropion.

52) This patient has paralytic ectropion with marked medial canthal tendon laxity.

A) *Aspergillus fumigatus*
B) *Candida* spp
C) *Acanthamoeba*
D) *Microspora* spp
E) *Onchocerca volvulus*
F) *Streptococcus viridans*
G) *Haemophilus influenza*
H) *Pseudomonas aeruginosa*
I) Herpes simplex
J) *Staphyloccus aureus*

Select the most likely organism for the each situation.

53) A 28-year-old presents with a history of unilateral gradual blurring and red eye. He has just returned from jungle trekking in a tropical country where he sustained a tree branch injury to his eye. There is an infiltrate on the cornea.

54) A patient who had a penetrating keratoplasty one year ago has a white branching lesion on the graft. However, he is uncomplaining and the eye is quiet. He has been on low dose topical steroid.

There are only 9 options for this question

A) Babies born before 27 weeks gestational age
B) Babies born between 27 and 32 weeks gestational age
C) Babies more than 32 weeks gestational age but with birthweight <1501 grams
D) Babies more than 32 weeks gestational age with birthweight > 1501 grams
E) The retinal vessels end in zone I or posterior zone II
F) There is plus disease
G) There is pre-plus disease
H) There is stage 3 disease in any zone
I) Stage 2 disease in zone 2

Select the most appropriate scenario for the each screening.

55) The first retinopathy of prematurity (ROP) screening examination should be undertaken at 30 to 31 weeks postmenstrual age.

56) The minimum frequency of ROP screening examination should be two weekly.

A) Optic disc drusen
B) Non-arteritic anterior ischaemic optic neuropathy
C) Arteritic anterior ischaemic optic neuropathy
D) Optic neuritis
E) Neuromyelitis optica
F) Idiopathic intracranial hypertension
G) Giant cell arteritis
H) Neuroretinitis
I) Optic nerve infiltrate
J) Astrocytoma

Select the likely diagnosis for each patient.

57) A 70-year-old presents with blurry vision in one eye. She complains of nocturnal sweats, shoulder stiffness and pain which last for an hour in the morning. She has been taking twice as long to finish her meals recently. The ESR is 30 and CRP 36.

58) A 40-year-old presents with left visual loss and periocular pain. The optic disc is swollen. She has weakness and numbness in her lower limbs. Lumbar puncture revealed elevated total protein levels and pleocytosis. There was no oligoclonal band. The MRI brain was normal. Spinal cord MRI showed contiguous signal abnormality over 3 vertebral segments.

A) Right superior rectus and inferior oblique weakening
B) Right inferior rectus resection
C) Right inferior oblique and left inferior rectus weakening
D) Right inferior oblique weakening
E) Right superior oblique tuck
F) Right medial rectus recession
G) Right medial rectus recession and lateral rectus resection
H) Left lateral rectus resection
I) Bilateral medial recti recessions
J) Bilateral lateral recti resections

Select the most appropriate procedure for the conditions mentioned.

59) A patient with Duane syndrome type 1 and a 25PD distant esotropia.

60) A 45-year-old with an acquired vertical diplopia and marked head tilt to the left. The right hypermetropia measures at 25PD in the primary position and is worse on looking left.

A) Amiloride
B) Atenolol
C) Bendrofluamethiazide
D) Furosemide
E) Ramipril
F) Spironolactone
G) Simvastatin
H) Sodium valproate
I) Sumatriptan
J) Topiramate

Select the likely drug which relates to the side-effect mentioned.

61) Hypokalaemia

62) Acute angle-closure glaucoma

There are only 9 options for this question

A) 0^0
B) 30^0
C) 45^0
D) 60^0
E) 90^0
F) 120^0
G) 135^0
H) 150^0
I) 180^0

Select the most appropriate answer for the following scenario.

63) The keratometry readings for a patient due for his cataract operation:

     K1 43.25@30

     K2 44.25@120

Where the main incision should be placed to reduce the amount of corneal astigmatism?

64) A patient who has less than 0.5DC of corneal astigmatism had a complicated cataract operation. The surgeon performed an extracapsular cataract extraction at the superior position and tightened the suture more than usual at the end of the operation. Where is the axis of the negative cylinder?

A) Lymphocytes
B) Eosinophils
C) Langhans cells
D) Touton cells
E) Epithelioid cells
F) Tubulofilamentour intranuclear inclusion in skeletal muscle
G) Ragged red fibre in skeletal muscle
H) Langerhan cells
I) Schaumann's bodies
J) Cowdry type A bodies

Select the likely histological findings for the each patient.

65) An 11-year-old presents with recurrent spontaneous hyphaema. He has multiple yellow papules on his skin.

66) A French-Canadian presents with diplopia in all direction of gaze and difficulty in swallowing. She has been suffering with proximal muscle weakness.

A) Multiple sclerosis
B) Acute disseminated encephalomyelitis
C) Myotonic dystrophy
D) Myasthenia gravis
E) Friedreich ataxia
F) Louis-Bar syndrome
G) Sturge-Weber syndrome
H) Parkinson's disease
I) von Reckinghausen disease
J) Neurofibromatosis type 2

Select the most appropriate diagnosis for the presentations mentioned

67) A teenager has been having difficulty in walking for the past few months. There is lower limb muscle wasting and weakness. The reflexes are absent and the plantar responses are up-going. The vibration and joint position sense are absent. He has nystagmus and pigmentary retinopathy.

68) A teenager complains of blurred and distorted vision. He has a slate grey lesion adjacent to a distorted optic disc. The associated retinal vessels are tortuous with a web of overlying gliosis. There is a strong family history of hearing loss and skin lesions.

A) Alport syndrome
B) Cogan syndrome
C) Cogan dystrophy
D) Fabry disease
E) Patau syndrome
F) Wilson disease
G) Labrador keratopathy
H) Salzmann nodular degeneration
I) Reis-Buckler dystrophy
J) Schnyder dystrophy

Select the most likely diagnosis for each patient.

69) A 10-year-old has partial hearing loss, abnormal renal function, and poor vision. Slit-lamp examination reveals posterior polymorphous dystrophy and peripheral retina flecks. His two brothers also have the same conditions.

70) A 22-year-old presents with a red, painful and photophobic eye. His also complains of worsening unilateral hearing defect and dizziness.

A) ETDRS
B) UKPDS
C) DRVS
D) DRS
E) DCCT
F) EMGT
G) AGIS
H) OHTS
I) CIGT
J) NTGS

Select the appropriate landmark study for each description.

71) Blood sugar level of less than 7mmol and blood pressure of less than 140/80mmHg reduce eye disease by a quarter and nephropathy by a third in type 2 diabetic patients.

72) The trabeculectomy group had more visual field and visual acuity loss compare to the medical treated group in the first 3 years. However these differences were not statistically significant in years 4 and 5 of follow-up.

A) Chandler syndrome
B) Axenfeld-Rieger syndrome
C) Iridoschisis glaucoma
D) Aniridia
E) Fuchs heterochromic cyclitis
F) Ghost cell glaucoma
G) Angle recession glaucoma
H) Haemolytic glaucoma
I) Cyclodialysis cleft
J) Pigment dispersion glaucoma

Select the likely type of glaucoma for each patient.

73) A patient in her 30's complains of decreased vision and occasional haloes. There is corneal, oedema, mild iris atrophy and broad based peripheral strands at the iridocorneal angle. The IOP is 45mmHg. The fellow eye is normal.

74) A young gentleman presented with an IOP of 50mmHg in the left eye. He sustained a blunt trauma in the eye 2 years ago. Gonioscopy revealed irregular widening of the ciliary body temporally and pigments scattered at the inferior angle and on the corneal endothelium.

A) Angiotensin-converting enzyme
B) Antinuclear antibody
C) Proteinase 3 ANCA
D) Myeloperoxidase ANCA
E) Skin pathergy test
F) Rheumatoid factor
G) Sabin-Feldman dye test
H) Tzanck smear
I) Anti-Ro antiboby
J) HLA-B27

Select the most useful test for each patient.

75) A patient with recurrent oral and genital ulceration presents with unilateral anterior uveitis.

76) A patient with myalgia and lymphadenopathy presents with unilateral chorioretinitis. Blood tests reveal deranged liver function test.

A) Adie tonic pupil
B) Argyll-Robertson pupil
C) Marcus Gunn pupil
D) Hutchison pupil
E) Third nerve palsy
F) Traumatic mydriasis
G) Pharmacological mydriasis
H) Central Horner syndrome
I) Preganglionic Horner syndrome
J) Postganglionic Horner syndrome

Select the likely cause of the pupil abnormalities.

77) A 35-year-old presents with recurrent unilateral temporal headache and periocular pain. The pain is sharp, lasting up to an hour. The nose is congested during an attack. He has anisocoria, and ptosis on the same side of the pain. The MRI head arranged by the GP was unremarkable.

78) A 75-year-old diabetic was referred for cataract operation. He has asymmetrical poor pupillary light reactions. However, both pupils constrict briskly to near stimuli. Dilatation with tropicamide was poor.

A) 50kHz
B) 500kHz
C) 1MHz
D) 10MHz
E) 20MHz
F) 50MHz
G) 100MHz
H) 200MHz
I) 1GHz
J) 3GHz

Select the most suitable ultrasonic frequency for the each scenario.

79) A patient with traumatic vitreous haemorrhage and very poor fundal view.

80) A 30-year-old patient with normal central anterior chamber depth presents with raised IOP a week after peripheral iridotomy.

A) Best vitelliform dystrophy
B) Sorsby pseudo-inflammatory macular dystrophy
C) Retinitis pigmentosa
D) Dry age related macular degeneration
E) X-linked retinoschisis
F) Stargardt disease
G) Fundus flavimaculatus
H) Leber congenital amaurosis
I) Malattia levantinese
J) Tay-Sachs disease

Select the likely diagnosis for the electrodiagnostic test outcomes.

81) A normal a-wave and marked attenuation of b-wave in the scotopic and photopic ERG.

82) The ERG is normal however the EOG light rise is subnormal.

A) Ventral midbrain fascicle near the cerebral peduncle
B) Red nucleus
C) Superior cerebellar peduncle
D) Superior colliculus
E) Inferior colliculus
F) Upper pons
G) Lower pons
H) Petrous apex
I) Cavernous sinus
J) Orbital apex

Select the likely anatomical site involved in the each case.

83) A 65-year-old presents with ipsilateral third nerve palsy, contralateral hemitremor and ataxia.

84) A 50-year-old was diagnosed with otitis media by the ENT surgeon. She presents a day later with right sided facial pain and weakness. She has limited abduction of the right eye.

A) Maxillary, zygomatic and palatine bones
B) Maxillary and zygomatic bones
C) Maxillary bone
D) Zygomatic and palatine bones
E) Palatine, greater wing of the sphenoid, maxillary and zygomatic bones
F) Ethmoidal, palatine and greater wing of the sphenoid bones
G) Frontal, palatine and ethmoidal bones
H) Ethmoidal, palatine and lacrimal bones
I) Maxillary, ethmoidal and lacrimal bones
J) Maxillary, lesser wing of the sphenoid and palatine bones

Select the bones that make up the aspect of the orbital wall.

85) Orbital floor

86) Medial orbital wall

A) A cluster of hard exudates 700µm away from the centre of the macular
B) Microaneurysm within 250µm from the centre of the macular
C) Capillary drop out (on the fundus angiogram) 250µm from the centre of the macular
D) Hard exudates 250µm away from the centre of the macular
E) Half a disc area of diffuse oedema at the centre of the macula
F) An eight months pregnant patient with moderate NPDR
G) Wide spread cotton wool spots
H) Early intraretinal microvascular abnormalities
I) A well controlled type 1 diabetic patient with a non-bleeding NVD < ¼ disc diameter
J) A well controlled type 2 diabetic patient with a non-bleeding NVD < ¼ disc diameter

Select the appropriate indication for argon laser treatment based on the ETDRS recommendations.

87) Modified macular grid laser

88) Panretinal photocoagulation

A) α1 – agonist
B) α2 – agonist
C) β1 - antagonist
D) β2 – antagonist
E) Non-selective β antagonist
F) Carbonic anhydrase inhibitor
G) Parasympathomimetic
H) F2-α prostaglandin analogue
I) Synthetic prostamide analogue
J) Cholinesterase inhibitor

Select the appropriate classification for each topical drug.

89) Brimonidine

90) Bimatoprost

EMQ Paper 1 Answers

1. H. Alport syndrome. Juvenile retinoschisis, blue-cone monochromatism, Schubert-Bornschein and Lowe syndrome are X-linked recessive. Aicardi syndrome is another X-linked dominant condition.

2. J. Sorsby retinopathy. Leber congenital amaurosis and gyrate atrophy are autosomal recessive. Leber optic neuropathy and Kearn-Sayre syndrome are mitochondrial inheritance disorders. A similar question was asked in the September 2010 EMQ paper. Learning the inheritance pattern of esoteric conditions may be a challenge, and revisiting the list may be best left until closer to the exam day.

3. D. Polyarteritis nodosa. This condition and antiphospholipid syndrome cause livedo reticularis

4. F. Wegener granulomatosis. Inflammatory bowel disease and rheumatoid arthritis can also cause this skin condition.

5. A. Chloramphenicol, which is a bacteriostatic.

6. H. Ofloxacin is bactericidal. Tetracycline and aminoglycoside (gentamicin) binds to 30S ribosomal subunit causing mRNA misreading; penicillin, amoxicillin, cephalosporin (cefradine) and vancomycin inhibit peptidoglycan synthesis of bacterial cell wall; fusidic acid inactivates enolpyruvyl transferase, thereby blocking cell wall synthesis; trimethoprim inhibits folate synthesis which is essential for cell wall synthesis.

7. C. Bilateral optic nerve glioma is associated with von Recklinghausen disease. This condition is inherited autosomal dominantly. The cutaneous lesions are cafe-au-lait spots and neurofibromas.

8. G. The most likely diagnosis is orbital myositis. The presentation is similar to orbital cellulitis however the normal white blood count and temperature are suggestive of a non-infective origin. In rhabdomyosarcoma, the presentation is usually earlier than this age. There is usually lid erythema despite the skin is not warm to touch.

9. D. Acethycholine (miochol) acts on all sympathetic and parasympathetic autonomic ganglia, and parasympathetic peripheral nerve endings. It has a very short half-life, however a fast onset of action. It is normally used to produce miosis in cataract surgery, which lasts approximately 20 minutes.

10. C. Guanethidine is a sympatholytic, which also increases outflow and reduces aqueous production. Physostigmine and ecothiopate are parasympathomimetic. Pilocarpine is a direct muscarinic. Cyclopentolate, tropicamide and atropine are competitive parasysmpatholytic acting at the post-synaptic cell membrane.

11. D. CMV retinitis is an opportunistic infection which usually affects HIV patients when the CD4+ count is fewer than 50cells/μl. Aspergillosis, tuberculosis, herpes simplex and herpes zoster related infections usually manifest when the CD4+ count is between 200 to 500cells/μl. Toxoplasma retinitis is another opportunistic disease which presents when the CD4+ count is below 200cells/μl.

12. J. Sicca syndrome can present when the CD4+ is about 700 or higher.

13. I. Patient on allopurinol requires a reduced dose of azathioprine. Mycophenolate is also a purine-antagonist however its effect is not affected by allopurinol.

14. A. Ciclosporin can also cause other gastrointestinal side-effects e.g. nausea, vomiting, abdominal pain and diarrhoea.

15. G. The angle for near remains significantly less than that for distance with +3.0D lenses (to interrupt accommodative convergence). Alternatively one eye is occluded for 30 minutes before the measurement is taken (to interrupt fusional convergence).

16. C. Esotropia is reduced but not completed eliminated by the correction of hypermetropia (unlike fully accommodative esotropia). Amblyopia and anisometropia are common.

17. B. This is Duane syndrome type 2.

18. G. About half the patients with Mobius syndrome have horizontal gaze palsy. The other half has bilateral sixth nerve palsy. The vertical gaze is usually preserved to a greater extend. The Bell's phenomenon in congenital fibrosis of the extraocular muscles patients is usually diminished or absent.

19. B. The long-standing bullous retinal dialysis requires draining and buckling to achieve satisfactory attachment of the retinal. A pars plana vitrectomy with silicone oil will almost invariably induce a cataract. Despite the latter can be removed eventually, the patient is unlikely to be pleased with the premature loss of accommodation.

20. G. 12% of C_3F_8 is likely to provide tamponade to the macular for the required duration in an upright position. 20% of SF_6 is unlikely to provide adequate tamponade for long. The other gas concentrations will cause an expansion of the gas volume which is dangerous to the

eye. Silicone oil is unnecessary since the patient will require another operation to remove the oil and there is likely to be more side-effects.

21. B. The NICE recommends β-blocker for patient younger than 60 year-old with an IOP 26-32 mmHg and cornea thickness of 555-590μm.

22. I. This patient has a low risk of conversion to glaucoma. The patient should be reviewed 12-24 months. The NICE guidelines also recommend the patient to be discharged after 3-5 years if there is no charge in the clinical findings.

23. C. The age of presentation and normal fundus suggest Stargardt disease. The presentation is usually in the first two decades of life and the prognosis is poor.

24. H. In enhanced S-cone syndrome, there is hyperfunction of the S-cones (short wavelength) which manifests as increased sensitivity to blue light. The L- and M-cone functions are impaired to a varying degree. The rod function is usually severely affected. Patients presents with nyctalopia in childhood and hemeralopia. Some patients have nummular hyperpigmentation at the mid-periphery of the retina.

25. B. Amorphous hyaline are deposited as granular lesions in the stroma and is stained bright red with Masson trichrome.

26. G. Mucopolysaccharidoses are a group of metabolic disorders caused by the absence or malfunctioning of lysosomal enzymes needed to break down glycosaminoglycans. The latter accumulates in various organs in the body. Scheie (and Hurler) has the most severe keratopathy and pigmentary retinopathy. Mental retardation occurs in Hurler and Sanfilippo. Scheie syndrome patients have normal life span and normal intelligence. Morquio and Maroteaux-Lamy are not associated with pigmentary retinopathy but mild corneal clouding and optic atrophy. Hunter and Sanfillippo have deafness and retinal degeneration but no corneal deposit.

27. F. Graves disease

28. G. Temporal arteritis. Asthma, anaphylaxis and penicillin allergy are Type I reactions. Polyarteritis nodosa, Wegener granulomatosis and systemic lupus erythematosus are Type III reactions. Marginal keratitis is caused by bacterial exotoxin, therefore is not a type of hypersensitivity.

29. I. -1.50 / +2.00 X 90

30. A. -3.00 / -1.50 X 135

31. C. Trauma is the most common cause of a direct carotid-cavernous fistula. Chemosis, dilated episcleral vessels, proptosis and an audible bruit are features highly suggestive of this condition. The sixth nerve is commonly affected due to its vulnerable position within the cavernous sinus.

32. J. Trapdoor fractures are more common in children due to the associated bone elasticity. The bone is more likely to bend and fracture in a linear pattern. Entrapment of muscle and soft tissue not only limit ocular motility but can cause ischemia. This may lead to subsequent loss of muscle function and permanent gaze restriction. Oculocardiac reflex can also occur. Surgical repair within a few days is required to achieve a good outcome.

33. C) Nothangel syndrome involves the superior cerebellar peduncle and the third nerve fasciculus. The former causes cerebellar syndrome. The most common causes for Nothangel syndrome are vascular lesion and tumour.

34. F. Acoustic neuroma usually presents with sensorineural hearing loss first. The patient's symptoms suggest ipsilateral V, VI, VII and VIII nerve palsy. Foville syndrome also includes central Horner syndrome which was not mentioned in his history.

35. C. PRP and intracameral bevacizumab provide better result compare to PRP alone. The raised IOP should be treated due to the already established vein occlusion. PRP and intracameral bevacizumab should be repeated if there is no regression of the rubeosis. Cyclodiode should be reserved for poorly controlled IOP.

36. G. The results of Central Retinal Vein Occlusion Study showed macular grid laser reduced the severity of angiographic macular oedema but did not improve the visual acuity compared to the control group. However, a trend in favour of treatment has been observed in younger patients. The treatment options available for this patient include intravitreal bevacizumab, ranibizumab and dexamethasone 0.7g intraocular implant. The triamcinolone acetonide available in the UK is not the same product, Trivaris, used in the SCORE-CRVO study, which is preservative free. There is no robust evidence to suggest Kenalog works as well as Trivaris.

37. B. This patient has Wilson's disease. This metabolic disorder causes copper to be deposited in the basal ganglia (causing dementia and rigidity), liver (causing jaundice) and Descemet's membrane (Kayser-Fleischer ring).

38. G. Galactosaemia classically causes oil droplet cataract within a few days of birth in majority of patients.

39. B. Neisseria species is the only gram negative diplococci. Knowledge of bacteria group provides a good guide to antibiotic choice before the culture sensitivity is available.

40. G. This is the most common pathogen in acute postoperative endophthalmitis. Staphylococcus aureus is coagulase positive.

41. D. Based on the statement given, the groups are presumed to be unpaired. The mean IOP in each group is distributed in a Gaussian fashion. The most appropriate test is the unpaired *t* test. For non-Gaussian distribution, the Wilcoxon test is used if the groups are paired, and the Mann-Whitney test for unpaired groups. For comparison of three or more groups in non-Gaussian population, Friedman test is employed for matched groups, and Kruskal-Wallis test for unmatched groups.

42. I. Pearson correlation is the most appropriate test to quantify the association between these two variables which are presumed to follow a Gaussian distribution. Spearman correlation is the equivalent for non-Gaussian distribution.

43. A. The symptoms suggest this patient has a craniopharyngioma. A growing lesion will initially compress on the chiasm superiorly and posteriorly, damaging the upper nasal fibres. The results in a bilateral inferotemporal field defect. As the lesion enlarges, a bitemporal hemianopia develops.

44. I. The signs constitute Gerstmann syndrome, which occur with dominant parietal lobe lesion. The patient is right handed therefore the left lobe is dominant.

45. C. T2 weighted MRI allows evaluation of 'activity' in the extraocular muscle in thyroid eye disease. The STIR suppresses orbital fat and is excellent for delineating adjacent structures.

46. J. Dacryoscintigraphy provides functional rather than anatomical information. The technique is non-invasive and sensitive. Unlike in a contrast dacryocystogram, no pressure is required to inject the contrast through the inferior canaliculus which may overcome any functional occlusion. Thus a normal dacryocystogram does not provide information related to functional obstruction. If a dacryoscintigram is normal, further investigation with dacryocystogram is unnecessary. In CT and MR dacryocystography, the contrast is instilled topically on the conjunctiva rather than

injected through the inferior canaliculus. The anatomical details are good in both methods however the functional data less so.

47. A. APMPPE usually affects young patients following a prodromal viral illness. Less commonly, patients have erythema nodosum and gastrointestinal symptoms. The condition usually affects both eyes despite the lesions may manifest in one eye first. The lesions cause a typical 'early block and late stain' pattern on fundus fluorescein angiography.

48. G. AZOOR is the most likely diagnosis. The visual field defect in AIBSES is demonstrated by an enlarged blind spot on the visual field test which is not the case here. FFA is usually normal in AZOOR. The ERG and EOG are helpful in the diagnosis of AZOOR. Despite the retinal dysfunction in AZOOR is focal clinically, ERG changes usually suggest a global deficit. Literature suggests multifocal ERG is sensitive in detecting areas of affected retina which correspond to the visual field defect.

49. H. SUSTAIN.

50. D. MARINA. ANCHOR trial looked at predominantly classic choroidal neovascularisation. MARINA and ANCHOR are two of the earliest landmark studies supporting the use of ranibizumab. PIER and EXCITE trials assessed the visual outcome of monthly ranibizumab injection for the first 3 months followed by quarterly dosing. The improvement of visual acuity was not comparable to ANCHOR or MARINA. PrONTO suggested a flexible dosing regimen with OCT-measured central thickness and visual acuity used as guiding criteria for re-treatment may be as effective as monthly dosing. FOCUS showed the visual outcome of combination of PDT and ranibizumab was not as good as ranibizumab alone. Pegaptanib was assessed in the VISION trial and PDT in VIP. The primary outcome in SAILOR was the incidence of serious adverse events in patients treated with repeated ranibizumab.

51. B. The Quickert sutures will evert the lid margin and the lateral tarsal strip tightens the horizontal laxity. Lower lid wedge resection would address the latter however not the entropion.

52. H. Medial canthal resection. The horizontal lid is shortened medially. In this procedure the inferior canaliculus is excised with the lid resection and marsupialised into the conjunctival sac.

53. A. Filamentous fungi such as *Aspergillus* spp and *Fusarium* spp are common pathogens in the tropical climate. The infiltrate typically has an indistinct margin associated with satellite lesions.

54. F. Infectious crystalline keratitis is an indolent infection associated with chronic use of topical steroid. *S. viridians* is the most common organism although other bacteria have been isolated.

55. A. This is based on the UK ROP Guideline published in 2008.

56. I. The minimum frequencies of screening should be weekly when the retinal vessels end in zone 1 or posterior zone II; or there is any plus or pre-plus disease or any stage 3 disease in any zone. In all other circumstances the screening should be fortnightly until the criteria for termination have been reached.

57. G. The nocturnal sweats and shoulder stiffness are suggestive of polymyalgia rheumatica. A limb girdle pattern can also occur, and the stiffness is worse in the morning. The clinical history is usually diagnostic. Despite the ESR is normal, the CRP is elevated. According to the literature, ESR can be normal in up to 17% of confirmed giant cell arteritis cases. The CRP is more sensitive and the combination of both has an increased sensitivity of 97-99%.

58. E. The majority of neuromylitis optica patients have opticomyelitis symptoms. One of the main distinctions from MS is NMO affects ≥3 vertebral segments of the spinal cord. Oligoclonal band is usually absent in CSF, and even when detected, tend to disappear with time. Serum aquaporin-4 antibody is present in most cases and is a useful diagnostic marker.

59. F. This is a small degree of esotropia, and the recommended procedure is unilateral medial rectus recession. Larger deviation would require bilateral recession of the medial recti and even vertical recti transposition. Lateral rectus should not be resected because this will almost invariably increase the globe retraction.

60. C. This is a right superior oblique palsy with a large vertical deviation. It is unlikely to be corrected with a right superior oblique tuck or right inferior oblique weakening. The appropriate treatment is weakening the right inferior oblique and contralateral inferior rectus. Weakening the inferior oblique and superior rectus unilaterally is likely to cause a reduction in elevation.

61. C. General pharmacology question may be asked in the written exam. This question was asked in the September 2010 paper. The second stem of the same question was on the cause of renal failure.

62. J. Topiramate is used to treat epilepsy and as a prophylaxis for migraine. The onset of attack is not dose related and can occur within two weeks of starting the medication. Topiramate can also cause

acute myopia, scleritis, blepharospasm, oculogyric crisis and peri-orbital oedema.

63. F. The main incision should be placed at the steepest meridian.

64. I. Despite the incision was performed superiorly, a tight suture would induce a with-the-rule astigmatism. The axis of the negative cylinder is at 180^0.

65. D. This patient has juvenile xanthogranuloma. There is usually localised or diffuse yellow infiltrate on the iris which can bleed spontaneously. The cutaneous lesions have a tendency to regress. Touton cells are formed by fusion of epithelioid cells (macrophages) with nuclei surrounded by foamy cytoplasm. They are also found in Erdheim-Chester disease (or lipoid granulomatosis), tuberous xanthoma, liposarcoma and dermatofibroma.

66. F. Oculopharyngeal dystrophy is more prevalent in the French-Canadians. This condition is a cause for chronic progressive external ophthalmoplegia. Ragged red fibres (due to accumulation of mitochondria) are found in Kearns-Sayre syndrome. Langhans cell are seen in granulomatous conditions (TB, chalazion, sarcoidosis) and contains epithelioid cells (macrophages) arranged in horse-shoed shape. Langerhan's cell on the other hand is an antigen presenting cell in the epidermis. Schaumann's bodies are found in sarcoidosis and Cowdry type A bodies are cells infected with herpes simplex virus.

67. E. Friedreich ataxia is an autosomal recessive progressive degeneration of the dorsal root ganglia, spinocerebellar tracts, corticospinal tracts and cerebellar Purkinje cells. The onset is during teenage years. Survival is ominous and rarely exceeds 20 years from diagnosis. Thirty percent of the patients have optic atrophy. Patients often have some eye signs due to cerebellar dysfunction - ocular dysmetria (over-shooting), opsoclonus (rapid, involuntary, multivector eye movements), ocular flutter, horizontal gaze-evoked nystagmus and skew deviation.

68. J. The history and signs suggest neurofibromatosis type 2. The retinal lesion is a combined hamartomas of RPE and retina. Despite the name suggests abnormal proliferation of the RPE and retina only, very often there are other type of tissues involved e.g. vitreous and retinal vessel. The lesion is difficult to treat and the prognosis is poor.

69. A. Alport syndrome is an X-linked dominant condition. Male offspring is almost certain to manifest the condition. The renal dysfunction is secondary to abnormal glomerular basement

membrane (defective type IV collagen). The ophthalmic signs include megalocornea, corneal arcus and pigment dispersion.

70. C. Cogan syndrome is an autoimmune vasculitis which normally affects young adults. Patients frequently present with interstitial keratitis and otological conditions (tinnitus, vertigo, deafness). Hearing symptoms require urgent immunosuppression to prevent permanent hearing loss. Ten percent of patients may go on to develop polyarteritis nodosa. Cogan dystrophy is map-dot-fingerprint dystrophy.

71. B. The UKPDS looked at type 2 diabetic patients and the DCCT assessed type 1 patients only. The ETDRS evaluated the outcome of early macular laser treatment in clinically significant macular oedema, PRP in early proliferative diabetic retinopathy and the effect of aspirin on diabetic retinopathy. The DRVS showed early vitrectomy improved final visual outcome in diabetic retinopathy related vitreous haemorrhage. The DRS found PRP to half the visual loss in proliferative diabetic retinopathy.

72. I. The CIGT showed that the trabeculectomy group had more cataract extractions than the medical group. The quality of life results indicated that both groups were satisfied with their treatment. While the surgery group reported more local eye symptoms e.g. grittiness, most symptoms were not sustained beyond the first 2 years of follow-up. The conclusion was patients should be treated medically before surgically. The EMGT was the first trial to prove early lowering of IOP can prevent disease progression. A mean IOP reduction of 25% was associated with a 27% reduction in risk of disease progression. Each 1 mmHg lowering of IOP correlated to a 10% risk reduction. The OHTS showed the 5 year cumulative probability of developing POAG was 4.4% in the medication group and 9.5% in the observation group. Although this does not imply that all patients with elevated IOP should receive medication, clinicians should consider initiating treatment for individuals who are at moderate or high risk for developing POAG. In the NTGS a reduction of IOP by 30% reduces disease progression in normal tension glaucoma patients. However, more than a third did not have any progression without treatment. The AGIS found that initial trabeculectomy retarded the progression of glaucoma more effectively in Caucasians than Afro-Americans. Black patients with advanced glaucoma have better visual field preservation if started with argon trabeculoplasty than trabeculectomy while Caucasian patients have better outcome vice versa. However, this recommendation is inconsistent with current medical practice. The study also showed that maintenance of IOP at

less than 18mmHg resulted in stable visual fields throughout the 6-year study.

73. A. The likely diagnosis is Chandler syndrome. The condition presents with hammered-silver corneal endothelium and corneal oedema. Iris stromal atrophy is only absent in about 60% of patients. The other disorders of iridocorneal endothelial syndrome are progressive iris atrophy and Cogan-Reese syndrome. The underlying pathology is abnormal proliferation of endothelial cells. These cells acquire microvilli and migrate across the iridocorneal angle. The HSV has been implicated but there is no definite link. Unlike Axenfeld-Rieger syndrome, this condition is unilateral, the iris-strands are broad based and there is no anterior displacement of the Schwalbe line.

74. G. Angle recession is a tear between the longitudinal and circular ciliary fibres. Cyclodialysis is a tear between the ciliary body and sclera spur. Both conditions can cause raised IOP, however through different mechanisms. Angle recession glaucoma is caused by direct damage to the trabecular meshwork itself which may not be evident initially. A cyclodialysis cleft usually results in hypotony and the IOP only become raised when the cleft closes spontaneously or surgically.

75. E. The patient has Behcet disease. The international criteria for diagnosis require oral ulceration and two of the following: genital ulcers, uveitis, defined skin lesions (erythema nodosum, folliculitis, papulo-pustular lesions) or a positive skin pathergy test. A positive test is highly specific for Behcet disease, and is due to the formation of papule or pustule within 48 hours after a sterile needle prick.

76. G. Patients with toxoplasmosis usually present with lymphadenopathy, mainly in the head and neck. There may be pyrexia, myalgia and general lethargy. Occasionally there are more severe manifestations including hepatitis (in this case), pneumonia and myocarditis. The Sabin-Feldman test utilises live toxoplasma gondii to be exposed to the patient's blood serum. A positive test occurs when the patient anti-toxoplasma IgGs lyse the organism cell membrane.

77. J. The symptoms suggest cluster headache and can cause postganglionic Horner syndrome. The attacks occur in 'clusters' and patients can be symptom free for a long time in between. It's unusual to have cluster headache after the age of 60. During an episode, changes occur in the hypothalamus which subsequently activates the trigeminal pathway and autonomic system. The latter causes lacrimation and rhinorrhea. The recurrent attack usually occurs in the early hours of the morning.

78. B. This patient has Argyll-Robertson pupils. The condition is usually bilateral however is frequently asymmetrical and may be unilateral. The site of lesion is in the region of the rostral midbrain interfering with the light reflex fibres, sparing the near response fibres located more ventrally. A slow gradual constriction of the pupil on near effort with similar redilation on relaxing accommodation suggests Adie tonic pupil, whereas in this case points to Argyll-Robertson pupils.

79. B. This frequency of ultrasound probe provides the best retinal visualisation on the B-scan.

80. F. The patient has iris plateau syndrome. The 50MHz probe is used for imaging of the iridocorneal angle. The probe uses higher frequency than posterior segment ultrasound providing greater resolution but lower tissue penetration. For general surgery and obstetrics, the ultrasound frequency is usually 5-6MHz.

81. E. The pattern describes the so called negative ERG. This is a result of disrupt communication between the photoreceptors and bipolar cells. Other conditions which can give rise to this appearance include congenital stationary night blindness (usually in scotopic ERG initially) and retinal vascular occlusions.

82. A. The EOG is a tedious test to perform, and the fact that most conditions which affect the ERG will also reduce the EOG light rise limit its use. However, it is particular helpful in Best vitelliform dystrophy where the light rise is consistently abnormal while the ERG is usually unaffected. The reason for this exceptional combination lays in the bestrophin gene which codes for a chloride channel protein in the RPE. Defect in the protein results in reduced conductivity and therefore reduced EOG light rise.

83. B. The signs are suggestive of Benedikt syndrome. The lesion involves the dorsal fascicle as it passes through the red nucleus. Weber syndrome is due to defect in the ventral fascicle near the cerebral peduncle and Nothangel syndrome the superior cerebellar peduncle. Superior colliculus is the region of the third nerve nuclear complex, and inferior colliculus fourth nerve nucleus.

84. H. The patient has Gradenigo syndrome which is usually triggered by localised inflammation or abscess of petrous apex. The sixth nerve is vulnerable due to its contact with the tip of the petrous pyramid. A careful identification of the neurological signs with concurrent sixth nerve palsy provides information on the likely pathological site. For example, contralateral hemiparesis suggests pontine lesion, ophthalmic branch of the trigeminal nerve involvement points to a

cavernous sinus lesion and third and fourth nerves palsy indicate orbital syndrome.

85. A. The posteromedial part of the maxillary bone is the weakness part of the floor and is the area that is usually involved in an orbital floor flow-out fracture.

86. I. The lamina papyracea formed by the ethmoidal bone is the weakness part of the medial wall. It is perforated by many foramina for blood vessels and nerves. Therefore it is a common infection conduit (ethmoidal sinusitis) for orbital cellulitis.

87. E. This is classified as clinically significant macular oedema. The criteria are retinal oedema within 500μm of the centre of the macula; hard exudates within 500μm of the centre of the macula with associated retinal thickening; and retinal oedema one disc area (1500μm) or larger, within one disc diameter of the centre of the macula.

88. J. The ETDRS compared early PRP with deferral of treatment, defined as careful follow-up (4 monthly intervals) and prompt PRP if progression to high-risk PDR occurred. Although the study did not provide definitive guidelines, the ETDRS suggested that PRP should not be recommended for mild or moderate NPDR. When retinopathy is more severe, PRP should be considered and should not be delayed if the eye has reached the high-risk proliferative stage. If the patient cannot be followed closely or if there are associated medical conditions e.g. impending cataract surgery or pregnancy, then early PRP may be indicated. Additional analyses of visual outcome in ETDRS patients with severe NPDR to non-high-risk PDR suggest PRP is particularly appropriate for type 2 diabetics. The risk of severe vision loss or vitrectomy was reduced by 50% (2.5% vs. 5%, $P = 0.0001$) in patients with type 2 diabetes who were treated early compared with deferral until high-risk PDR developed. For type 1 diabetics, the timing of the PRP will depend on the compliance with follow-up and the status and response to treatment of the fellow eye.

89. B. Brimonidine is contraindicated in patient on monoamine oxidase inhibitor since it can potentiate a hypertensive crisis. Tricyclic antidepressants can blunt brimonidine IOP lowering effect. Apraclonidine is a partial α2–agonist

90. I. Latanoprost, tafluprost and travoprost are F2-α prostaglandin analogue. Bimatoprost is the only synthetic prostamide analogue.

MCQ Paper 1

1) Which type of hypersensitivity reaction is ocular cicatrical pemphigoid?
   a. I
   b. II
   c. III
   d. IV

2) Where on the eyelid is an epibulbar dermoid most commonly found?
   a. superiorly
   b. inferotemporally
   c. nasally
   d. superiotemporally

3) Which layer of the cornea does the calcium precipitate in band keratopathy?
   a. epithelium
   b. Bowman
   c. stroma
   d. Descemet

4) Below are the causes of interstitial keratitis except
   a. Leishmania
   b. Syphilis
   c. Brucellosis
   d. Loaisis

5) Hutchinson's triad refers to the signs below except
   a. saddle nose
   b. interstitial keratitis
   c. notched teeth
   d. sensorineural deafness

6) Ocular associations with retinitis pigmentosa are listed below except
   a. optic disc drusen
   b. myopia
   c. intermediate uveitis
   d. nuclear sclerosis

7) Stimulation of adrenergic receptor causes
   a. significant ciliary muscle relaxation
   b. decreased aqueous outflow
   c. contraction of Muller's muscle
   d. dilatation of conjunctival vessels

8) Congenital toxoplasmosis causes the conditions below except
   a. optic neuropathy
   b. hydrocephalus
   c. intracranial calcification
   d. retinochoroiditis

9) The image of a convex mirror is not
   a. erect
   b. diminished
   c. virtual
   d. real

10) If the red Maddox rod is in front of the right eye and the patient sees the red line below the white dot, this indicates
   a. right hypotropia
   b. left hypotropia
   c. right exotropia
   d. horizontal orthophoria

11) The spherical aberration in the eye is reduced by the following except
   a. the anterior corneal surface is flatter peripherally than at its centre
   b. the nucleus of the lens of the eye has a higher refractive index than the lens cortex
   c. the retina is a spherical surface
   d. retina cones are more sensitive to paraxial light than to oblique light through the peripheral cornea (Stiles-Crawford effect)

12) The statements below are true about Panum's space except
   a. Panum's area is as zone in front and behind of the horopter
   b. all objects stimulate corresponding retinal elements
   c. stereopsis exist in this space
   d. the Panum's area is wider in the periphery

13) The maximum level of horizontal Fresnel prism which could be worn without unacceptable adverse visual acuity is
   a. 10^0
   b. 40PD
   c. 30^0
   d. 50PD

14) Which statement about strabismus surgery is true?
   a. the inferior rectus is the shortest extraocular muscle
   b. lower eyelid retraction can occur after recession of more than 4mm of inferior rectus
   c. the lateral rectus has no intermuscular septum connection to the oblique muscles
   d. recession of superior rectus in the order of 10 mm is likely to significantly change the upper eyelid position

15) Which feature is true in nystagmus blockage syndrome?
   a. The nystagmus is absent when the eyes are closed
   b. The esotropia is due to access accommodation exerted
   c. Pupil mydriasis may occur during the esotropic phase
   d. The squinting eye remains adducted when a base-out prism is introduced in front of the fixing eye

16) The features of microtropia are listed below except
   a. foveal suppression scotoma is present in the affected eye
   b. abnormal binocular single vision with sensory and motor fusion
   c. stereopsis is usually absent
   d. anisometropia in the majority of cases

17) Which contralateral extraocular muscle is not affected as a result of third nerve palsy?
   a. lateral rectus
   b. superior rectus
   c. inferior rectus
   d. inferior oblique

18) Which cell does class II major histocompatibility complex activate?
   a. macrophages
   b. T cytotoxic cells
   c. B cells
   d. T helper cells

19) The power of a study is dependent on the factors below except
   a. size of the difference to be detected
   b. size of the study population
   c. significance level required
   d. standard deviation of the study

20) Which statement is true regarding visual electrophysiological test?
   a. a history of photogenic epilepsy is usually not contraindicated
   b. cardiac pacemakers or cochlear implants are unlikely to interfere with the recording
   c. it is important for the patient to wear the appropriate refractive correction
   d. pupil dilation is not required for EOG

21) The statements below are true about the ERG except
   a. processes that disrupt communication between the photoreceptors and bipolar cell characteristically reduce the amplitude of the a-wave
   b. the a-wave originates from the photoreceptors
   c. the 30Hz flicker contains contributions from both the on- and off-bipolar cells but not from the photoreceptors
   d. congenital stationary night blindness causes a 'negative ERG'

22) When should antiretroviral therapy be started based on the level of CD4+ count (cells/μl)?
 a. 100
 b. 250
 c. 350
 d. 500

23) The following eye structures are derived from surface ectoderm except
 a. lacrimal gland
 b. meibomian glands
 c. corneal epithelium
 d. orbital bones

24) Identify the gram positive bacterium.
 a. *Propionibacterium acnes*
 b. *Haemophilus influenza*
 c. *Pseudomonas aeroginosa*
 d. *Neisseria meningitides*

25) This human leucocyte antigen (HLA) is associated with birdshot retinochoroidopathy.
 a. HLA B27
 b. HLA A29
 c. HLA B51
 d. HLA A11

26) Which statement is true about the human retina?
 a. there are 10 times more rod than cones
 b. the fovea does not contain any rods
 c. the photoreceptors are supplied by the retinal arteries
 d. the retina is the thickest in the mid-periphery

27) Cataract usually occurs in the conditions below except
 a. hyperglycaemia
 b. secondary hypoglycaemia
 c. primary hyperparathyroidism
 d. hypoparathyroidism

28) The condition that can cause angle-closure glaucoma is
    a. corneal epithelial downgrowth
    b. Schwartz-Mazuo syndrome
    c. Fuch heterochronic cyclitis
    d. iridocorneal endothelial syndrome

29) The statements regarding retinopathy of prematurity are true except
    a. usually affects the temporal periphery first
    b. is not present at birth
    c. majority of active ROP patients develop cicatricial complications
    d. spontaneous regression can occur in partial retinal detachment

30) Which statement is true regarding posterior vitreous detachment?
    a. usually causes tobacco dusting in the anterior vitreous
    b. does not cause vitreous haemorrhage
    c. impedes the progression of diabetic retinopathy
    d. does not occur with trauma

31) It is illegal to drive in the United Kingdom if the patient has
    a. a reproducible cluster of 4 adjoining point defects partly within the central 20 degree area on the Estermann visual field test
    b. a reproducible cluster of 3 adjoining points missed along the horizontal meridian of the Estermann visual field test
    c. an recent inferior altitudinal defect in the better seeing eye
    d. severe night blindness

32) Which is contraindicated to FFA?
    a. breastfeeding
    b. shellfish allergy
    c. liver dysfunction
    d. pregnancy

33) The term which refers to the gain associated with the best alternative use of a healthcare resource is called
    a. contingency business plan
    b. healthcare economics
    c. alternative economics
    d. opportunity cost

34) The signs associated with anaphylactic shock are listed below except
   a. hypotension
   b. bradycardia
   c. vomiting
   d. rhinitis

35) According to the Royal College of Ophthalmologists preferred practice guidance on diabetic retinopathy, which group of patients should be referred to the ophthalmologists within 2 weeks?
   a. grade U
   b. grade M1
   c. grade R2
   d. grade R3

36) What is the percentage of severe visual loss within 2 years in a patient found to have severe neovascularisation of the disc (NVD) without vitreous haemorrhage?
   a.   15%
   b.   26%
   c.   37%
   d.   45%

37) Which structure in the orbit does the parasympathetic nerve travel on?
   a.   superior division of the third nerve
   b.   inferior division of the third nerve
   c.   the trochlear nerve
   d.   the nasociliary nerve

38) Posterior lenticonus is associated with
   a.   posterior polymorphous corneal dystrophy
   b.   keratoconus
   c.   irregular astigmatism
   d.   bilateral lens defect in most cases

39) The statements regarding the human cornea are true except
   a. the refractive indices of the Descemet membrane and the corneal endothelium are the same
   b. the Descemet membrane thicken with age
   c. obtains most of its nutrient from the limbal capillaries and tear
   d. corneal epithelium is freely permeable to lipid-soluble substance

40) A patient with neurofibromatosis type 2 has a child with the same condition from her previous marriage. She wants to know her chances of an affected offspring with her new partner who is healthy and does not a family history of the condition.
   a. 0%
   b. 25%
   c. 50%
   d. 100%

41) According to the National Institute for Health and Clinical Excellence (NICE) glaucoma management guideline 2009, how should a healthy 58-year-old patient with corneal thickness of 580μm, IOP of 27mmHg, normal optic disc and low risk factor for glaucoma be managed?
   a. treat with prostaglandin analogue
   b. treat with β-blocker
   c. monitor in 2 – 4 months
   d. discharged to his optician

42) Select the true statement regarding fluorescein angiography.
   a. the excitation peak for fluorescein is about 490nm
   b. the emission peak for fluorescein is about 580nm
   c. only yellow-green light is filtered into the eye
   d. the usual concentration of fluorescein is 35%

43) Which drug is a direct acting parasympathomimetic?
   a. pilocarpine
   b. physostigmine
   c. tropicamide
   d. cocaine

44) The following types of cell are involved in acute inflammation except
   a. T-lymphocytes
   b. neutrophils
   c. macrophages
   d. eosinophils

45) The advantages of CT scans compare to MRI scans are listed except
   a. less patient cooperation is needed
   b. visualisation of abnormal flow in blood vessels
   c. quicker
   d. excellent visualisation between muscles, orbital fat and bone

46) Select the true statement about β-blocker.
   a. selective β_1-blocker has minimal effect on the lungs
   b. β-blockers increases aqueous drainage
   c. non-selective β-blockers are equipotent at the β_1 and β_2 receptors
   d. tachyphylaxis occurs in 90% of patients on β-blocker

47) Which description is false about *toxoplasma gondii*?
   a. the chances of passing the infection to the foetus increases as the pregnancy progresses
   b. *toxoplasma gondii* is a protozoan
   c. acquired toxoplasmosis presents as meningoencephalitis in most patients
   d. *toxoplasma gondii* is an intracellular organism

48) The early stage of retrobulbar optic neuritis is usually associated with
   a. a pale disc
   b. swollen disc
   c. inferior altitudinal defect
   d. pain on ocular movement

49) Which of the following is incorrect?
   a. type I error is influenced by the false positive rate (α)
   b. type II error is influenced by the size of the sample
   c. the *p* value measures the probability that the null hypothesis is true
   d. the power of a test depends upon the size of the sample

50) Select the appropriate visual test for a healthy 3-month-old baby.
    a. Kay pictures
    b. forced preferential looking
    c. Sheridan-Gardner chart
    d. Cardiff acuity cards

51) The descriptions about Stickler syndrome are true except
    a. the condition is associated with Marfanoid habitus
    b. patients have Pierre Robin syndrome
    c. leads to progressive myopia
    d. inheritance is autosomal dominant

52) What procedure is appropriate for a 3-year-old child with congenital ptosis and levator function of 3mm?
    a. brow suspension with autologous fascia lata
    b. brow suspension with Mersilene mesh
    c. levator resection
    d. aponeurosis advancement

53) The B-scan characteristics of a choroidal melanoma are described below except
    a. choroidal excavation
    b. mushroom configuration
    c. high reflectivity
    d. orbital shadowing

54) Which combination makes up the 0.5D Jackson cross cylinder?
    a. +0.5DS/-1.00DC
    b. +1.00DS/-0.5DC
    c. -0.5DS/-0.5DC
    d. +0.5DS/-0.5DC

55) A 10-year-old patient has mild left esotropia. Her acuities are 6/6 OD and 6/9 OS. Which is unlikely to occur with the Worth four-dot test? (green filter OD and a red filter OS)
    a. she sees two green lights for distance fixation
    b. she sees all four lights for near fixation
    c. she sees two red lights for distance fixation with +5D lens OD
    d. she sees two red lights for near fixation

56) What is the minimal cornea thickness for LASIK refractive surgery?
   a. 250µm
   b. 350µm
   c. 450µm
   d. 550µm

57) Where is the standard reference plane taken in the Heidelberg retinal tomography of the optic disc?
   a. 50µm below the optic nerve head boundary line at the nasal disc edge along the horizontal midline
   b. 50µm below the optic nerve head boundary line at the temporal disc edge along the horizontal midline
   c. on the surface of the optic nerve head boundary line at the nasal disc edge along the horizontal midline
   d. on the surface of the optic nerve head boundary line at the temporal disc edge along the horizontal midline

58) Long term systemic steroid treatment can cause the following except
   a. hypertension
   b. hyperglycaemia
   c. osteoporosis
   d. hyperkalaemia

59) In hypothesis testing, β is the probability of committing a Type II error. Therefore $1 - \beta$ is
   a. the probability of rejecting the null hypothesis when the alternate hypothesis is true
   b. the probability of failing to reject the null hypothesis when the alternate hypothesis is true
   c. the probability of accepting the null hypothesis when the null hypothesis is true
   d. the probability of rejecting alternative hypothesis when null hypothesis is true

60) What is the probability of developing multiple sclerosis within 10 years if a patient presents with first episode of optic neuritis and the MRI brain shows T2 signal lesions but no clinical evidence of multiple sclerosis?
   a. 20%
   b. 38%
   c. 44%
   d. 56%

61) Which statement is incorrect about the OCT?
   a. OCT uses low coherence interferometry
   b. the basis of imaging depends on the contrast in optical reflectivity between different tissue structures
   c. thin retinal haemorrhage appears hyporeflective
   d. hard exudates is highly reflective

62) Which description is true about non-arteritic anterior ischaemic optic neuropathy?
   a. FFA shows leakage from the optic disc
   b. cotton wool spots are common
   c. visual acuity tend to improve with time
   d. there is an association with giant cell arteritis

63) The histology of this tumour shows cells with large hyperchromatic nuclei with vacuolated cytoplasm stained with Sudan black.
   a. squamous cell carcinoma
   b. sebaceous cell carcinoma
   c. basal cell carcinoma
   d. Merkel cell carcinoma

64) Neovascular glaucoma occurs with the following conditions except
   a. long standing retinal detachment
   b. choroidal melanoma
   c. branch retinal vein occlusion
   d. cavernous sinus thrombosis

65) Which is the most appropriate investigation for a patient suspected of demyelinating disease?
    a.   MRI with FLAIR sequence
    b.   MRI with STIR sequence
    c.   CT
    d.   MR angiography

66) A patient information can be disclosed to the appropriate third party without his/her consent in the following scenario except
    a.   recently diagnosed HIV positive
    b.   investigation into a healthcare professional's fitness to practise
    c.   requested by the police
    d.   if the safety of the patient's family members is at stake

67) Which statement does not apply to optic nerve hypoplasia?
    a.   can be bilateral or unilateral
    b.   the visual acuity is almost always impaired
    c.   the retinal blood vessels are of normal calibre
    d.   is linked with maternal diabetes

68) The listed conditions can cause exudative retinal detachment except
    a.   choroidal neovascularisation
    b.   panretinal photocoagulation
    c.   posterior scleritis
    d.   retinoschisis

69) Which statement regarding fluorescein angiography is incorrect?
    a.   the arteriovenous phase lasts for 1-2 seconds
    b.   the diameter of the retinal vessels visualised on a fluorescein angiogram is larger than that of a fundal photograph
    c.   the choroidal phase usually occurs within 5 seconds after dye injection
    d.   late staining of the optic disc is normal

70) Hypertension controlled by this medication has been shown to reduce the progression of diabetic retinopathy over 2 years.
    a. atenolol
    b. lisinopril
    c. amlodipine
    d. furosamide

71) Fungi are stained with the following except
    a. Grocott hexamine silver
    b. Gomori methanamine silver
    c. Giemsa
    d. Periodic acid-Schiff

72) Which statement associated with congenital cataract is true?
    a. unilateral cataracts are inherited autosomal recessively
    b. bilateral cataract is always associated with systemic disease
    c. the majority of congenital cataract is unilateral
    d. unilateral cataract usually affects full-term and healthy infants

73) An ophthalmologist has carried out a measurement of IOP on a random sample of 20 patients taking a new anti-glaucoma treatment and 20 patients not on treatment. A test of significance was performed with the appropriate null and alternative hypothesis. The p value was 0.03. Which statement is true?
    a. the result is statistically significant if the confidence level is set at 99%
    b. there is some reason to believe the null hypothesis may be false
    c. the probability of being incorrect is 3%
    d. only 3% of patients did not respond to the treatment

74) Which description is true regarding temporal arteritis?
    a. there is no specific clinical signs to diagnose temporal arteritis
    b. ESR has a higher sensitivity for temporal arteritis than CRP
    c. temporal artery biopsy is unhelpful after a week of starting systemic steroid
    d. the platelet count remains abnormal on steroid treatment

75) The following statements about contrast dacryocystography are true except
   a. the technique requires catheterisation of the inferior canaliculi
   b. ionising radiation used does reach the lenses
   c. good functional or physiological data are usually obtained
   d. an unsubtracted image is usually taken to demonstrate relevant bony detail

76) Which statement regarding juvenile idiopathic arthritis is true?
   a. the uveitis causes pain and conjunctival injection
   b. macular oedema is a cause of visual loss
   c. uveitis is uncommon in the pauciarticular group
   d. uveitis usually requires systemic steroid treatment

77) The descriptions about acetazolamide are true except
   a. increases the renal excretion of bicarbonate
   b. acts on the proximal convoluted renal tubules
   c. can cause hyponatraemia
   d. can cause metabolic alkalosis

78) Which statement is incorrect regarding wavefront aberrometry?
   a. the algorithm used to analyse the wavefront includes Zernicke polynomial
   b. the algorithm used to analyse the wavefront includes Fourier analysis
   c. higher-order aberrations cannot be removed from the wavefront map
   d. a pulse of infrared light is emitted into the eye

79) Select the appropriate histological stain for calcium.
   a. von Kossa
   b. Congo red
   c. Prussian blue
   d. Masson trichrome

80) According to the General Medical Council Good Medical Practice, a doctor should not
   a. advise patients on the effects of their life choices on their health
   b. provide non-urgent medical treatment to his mother
   c. try to resolve any patient safety issue himself initially
   d. give priority to investigation on the basis of clinical need

81) Which of the following statements is true?
   a. the p value measures the probability that the alternative hypothesis is true
   b. the p value measures the probability of making a type 2 error
   c. an extremely small p value indicates that the actual data differs markedly from that expected if the null hypothesis was true
   d. the larger the p value, the more likely the null hypothesis is false

82) What is the most common pathogen in delayed-onset postoperative endophthalmitis?
   a. *Propionibacterium acnes*
   b. *Staphylococcus epidermidis*
   c. *Streptococcus pneumonia*
   d. *Pseudomonas aeruginosa*

83) The patient has retinoblastoma. The parents, who are both healthy, would like to know the probability of having another child with retinoblasma.
   a. 2%
   b. 10%
   c. 25%
   d. 40%

84) Which statement is not true regarding infantile esotropia?
   a. it is associated with dissociated vertical deviation
   b. latent nystagmus is usually present
   c. patients with cross-fixation should have occlusion therapy
   d. the angle of deviation is similar for near and distance

85) Pars planitis can cause the conditions below except
   a. epiretinal membrane
   b. retinal detachment
   c. vitreous haemorrhage
   d. ischaemic maculopathy

86) Which statement regarding epiphora in a 6-month-old is incorrect?
   a. there is bilateral involvement in majority of the cases
   b. in majority of cases, it resolves spontaneously by 1 year of age
   c. the most common cause is a membranous obstruction of the distal end of the nasolacrimal duct
   d. it may be associated with hypertelorism

87) The side-effects of tropicamide includes the followings except
   a. gastrointestinal disturbance
   b. skin erythema
   c. bradycardia
   d. pyrexia

88) The indications for dacryocystography exclude
   a. suspected lacrimal sac tumour
   b. congenital craniofacial abnormality
   c. suspected dacryolith in a patient patent to lacrimal syringing
   d. suspected incomplete proximal canalicular obstruction

89) Increased IOP is a recognised feature of the listed conditions except
   a. juvenile idiopathic arthritis
   b. carotid-cavernous fistula
   c. thyroid eye disease
   d. idiopathic intracranial hypertension

90) According to the Royal College of Ophthalmologists guideline for screening and treatment of retinopathhy of prematurity, when should a baby born at week 26 gestational age be screened?
   a. between 2 to 3 weeks postnatal age
   b. between 5 to 6 weeks postnatal age
   c. at 30 to 31 weeks postmenstrual age
   d. at 32 to 33 weeks postmenstrual age

MCQ Paper 1 Answers

1) b. Type II hypersensitivity is a cytotoxic reaction. Other diseases caused by the same type of reaction include myasthenia gravis, Graves's disease, mucous membrane pemphigoid and Wegener granulomatosis.

2) b. As with coloboma, dermoid is most commonly found in the inferotemporal region.

3) b. The calcium salt is precipitated from tear into the Bowman's layer. Band keratopathy occurs with increasing age and is related to ocular (chronic uveitis, phthisis bulbi, silicone oil, alkali injury), systemic (hypercalcaemia, hyperphosphataemia, hyperuricaemia) and hereditary causes.

4) d. Loa loa does not cause cornea inflammation. Interstitial keratitis is a type IV hypersensitivity reaction. It is also caused by non-infectious factors e.g. sarcoidosis, lymphoma, contact-lens, Cogan's syndrome.

5) a. Saddle nose occurs in some patients with syphilis but is not part of the triad.

6) d. Posterior subcapsular sclerosis is common in all forms of RP and not nuclear sclerosis.

7) c. Adrenergic agonist causes elevation of ptosis due to adrenergic receptors on the Muller muscle. Adrenergic stimulation only causes slight ciliary muscle relaxation.

8) a. Congenital toxoplasmosis does not affect the optic nerve.

9) d. The image of a convex mirror is always erect, virtual and diminished. The image of a concave mirror is dependent of the distant from the mirror. If the object is more than twice the focal length, the image is diminished, inverted and real. If the object is between the focal length and the radius of the mirror, the image formed is enlarged, inverted and real. If the object is within the focal length, the image is enlarged, erect and virtual.

10) a. Right hypotropia. This is a crossed diplopia.

11) a. This feature reduces ocular oblique astigmatism and has no effect on spherical aberration.

12) a. Objects on the horopter line stimulate the corresponding retinal points. In the Panum's area, non-corresponding points are stimulated.

The disparity of information is used to produce a perception of binocular depth.

13) c. 30^0 can be applied to either eye but high-powered prisms may not be tolerated because of their adverse effect on visual acuity; usually up to 20^0 can be worn comfortably, at least by children.

14) b. The inferior rectus has a strong indirect attachment to the lower eyelid that can result in lower eyelid retraction after a recession of 4mm or more, especially in patients with thyroid eye disease who have pre-existing lid retraction. The strong intermuscular septum between the inferior rectus and inferior oblique (the Lockwood ligament) may be responsible for the increased incidence of posterior slippage of the inferior rectus. The medial rectus is the only muscle without an intermuscular septum connection to an oblique muscle, therefore if it 'slips' during surgery, it retracts posteriorly within its capsule and can be difficult to relocate.

15) d. The esotropia is due convergence mechanism hence the prism has little effect on the squinting eye. The nystagmus is present and remains the same whether both eyes are opened or if one is covered. It increases in intensity when the eye is abducted and is blocked when the eye is adducted. The esotropia is non-accommodative and variable. The patient adopts a face turn to the side of the fixing eye. (Note: patients with DVD adopt a head tilt to the side of the fixing eye). Amblyopia is common and the esotropia is usually unilateral. Pupil miosis may occur during the esotropic phase. Nystagmus blockage syndrome has a high association with neurological disorders, and ocular or oculocutaneous albinism. The result of strabismus surgery is unfortunately unpredictable.

16) c. Stereopsis is reduced however rarely absent. Microtropia is more prevalent in esotropia. It's classified into cases with or without identity. The former is said to present when the deviation is associated with eccentric fixation which is coincident with the angle of deviation. No manifest deviation is detected. The visual acuity is usually reduced and a binocular single vision is demonstrable. Microtropia without identity is present when a very small manifest deviation is seen (on cover test). The central / eccentric fixation is not coincident with the angle of deviation.

17) c. Third nerve palsy causes overaction of the contralateral extraocular muscles listed above except the inferior rectus. In order for the latter to occur, the ipsilateral superior oblique has to be affected.

18) d. T helper cells. Class II MHC is present in antigen-presenting cells only (e.g. macrophages, dendritic cells, B cells). Class I MHC is present in all nucleated cells and activates T cytotoxic cells only.

19) d. The power of a study is the probability of reducing type 2 error, in other words the probability of not accepting a false null hypothesis.

20) c. The pupils are required to be dilated for EOG and full-field ERG. A period of dark adaptation is also required. Although these tests avoid epileptogenic flash frequencies, a history of photogenic epilepsy is normally a contraindication to testing.

21) a. The b-wave is disrupted, which produces a 'negative ERG'. This occurs in X-linked retinoschisis, congenital stationary night blindness and retinal vascular occlusions.

22) c. The British HIV Association 2008 guideline recommends antiretroviral treatment to be started when the CD4+ count is ≤350.

23) d. The orbital bones are formed from neural crest cells. Surface ectoderm also forms the conjunctival epithelium, lacrimal drainage apparatus, eyelids, Moll and Zeis glands.

24) a. *Propionibacterium acnes* is a gram positive bacillus.

25) b. HLA B27 is associated with anterior uveitis and ankylosing spondylitis, HLA A11 sympathetic ophthalmia and HLA B51 Behcet disease.

26) b. The fovea is capillary and rod free. The human eye consists of about 120×10^6 rods and 6×10^6 cones. The retina is the thickest at the far periphery.

27) c. Cataract is not precipitated by primary hyperparathyroidism which causes hypercalcaemia. Secondary hyperparathyroidism causes hypocalcaemia.

28) d. ICE syndrome can cause open and closed angle glaucoma. The corneal endothelium grows over the trabecular meshwork causing obstruction and damage to the trabecular meshwork. Peripheral anterior synaechiae can develop and cause angle closure.

29) c. Only about 20% of infants with active ROP develop cicatricial complications. The remaining 80% regresses spontaneously. The CRYO-ROP study found 18% of babies below 1251g developed stage 3, with only 6% reaching threshold and requiring treatment.

30) c. Vitreous haemorrhage can be caused by a PVD without a retinal break.

31) a. For motor car drivers, the following are regarded as unacceptable:

   i. A cluster of 4 or more adjoining points that is either wholly or partly within the central 20 degree area

   ii. Loss of both a single cluster of 3 adjoining missed points up to and including 20 degrees from fixation, and any additional separate missed point(s) within the central 20 degree area

   iii. Any central loss that is an extension of a hemianopia or quadrantanopia of size greater than 3 missed points

32) a. Fluorescein does not contain iodine but indocyanine does. Shellfish allergy is not a contraindication to FFA, but iodide allergy is a relative contraindication. Breastfeeding is a contraindication since fluorescein is excreted in human milk. Renal impairment is also a contraindication.

33) d. The aim of economics is to ensure that the chosen activities have benefits which outweigh their opportunity costs or the most beneficial activities are chosen within the resources available.

34) b. Tachycardia is caused by the response to profound vasodilation.

35) d. Grade R2 and M1 patients should be seen within 13 weeks. Grade U is ungradeable (e.g. due to dense cataract, uncooperative patient).

36) b. A similar question was asked in the MCQ paper in September 2010. Mild NVD with haemorrhage carries a risk of 26% of severe visual loss (defined as 5/200) which is reduced to 4% with PRP; severe NVD without haemorrhage is also 26%, reduced to 9% with PRP; severe NVD with haemorrhage 37% reduced to 20% with PRP and severe NVE with haemorrhage 30% reduced to 7% with PRP. These figures are obtained from the ETDRS.

37) b. The parasympathetic nerves travel along the inferior division of oculomotor nerve and reach the ciliary ganglion via the nerve supplying the inferior oblique muscle continuing along the short ciliary nerve to innervate the sphincter pupillae.

38) c. Posterior lenticonus occurs sporadically and not associated with any systemic abnormalities. It is usually unilateral. The astigmatism is lenticular and not corneal.

39) c. Most of the nutrients are supplied by the aqueous and only about 10% by the tear film and limbal vessels.

40) c. Both types of neurofibromatosis are inherited in an autosomal dominant fashion.

41) b. According to the recommendations, patients with cornel thickness 555 - 590μm, IOP 26 - 32mmHg and age up to 60 should be considered for topical β-blocker treatment.

42) a. The emission peak of fluorescein is 530nm. White light is filtered and the emerging blue light enters the eye to excite the fluorescein molecule circulating in the fundus. Yellow-green light is emitted and another filter is in place to block any reflected blue light passing into the camera. The usual concentration of fluorescein is 10%. Up to 25% can be used for eye with opaque media.

43) a. Physostigmine (treatment for *Phthirus pubis*) is a cholinesterase inhibitor (an indirect acting parasympathomimetic). Tropicamide is a competitive parasysmpatholytic acting at the post-synaptic cell membrane. Cocaine is an indirect acting sympathomimetic, and inhibits the reuptake of catecholamines and causes partial cycloplegia.

44) a. T-lymphocytes are seen in chronic inflammatory reaction.

45) b. MRI is able to detect abnormal flow in blood vessels. CT scans optimally demonstrates bony structures including erosion, scalloping and bone defects. It is the investigation of choice for preseptal cellulitis and dermoid cyst.

46) c. Non-selective β-blockers have the same effect on β_1 and β_2 receptors. Despite β_1-blocker has less effect on the lung bronchioles, its use is still contraindicated in severe asthmatic patients.

47) c. Most patients with acquired toxoplasmosis are subclinical, and in minority of the patients it can present as generalised lymphadenopathy and meningoencephalitis. In immunocompromised patients, it may present as an intracranial mass. There is a higher chance of passing the infection to the foetus as the pregnancy progresses; however the severity of the disease is usually less serious. If the mother is infected before the pregnancy, the chances are remote, in the first trimester 15% and the third trimester up to 40%.

48) d. In the acute stage of retrobulbar neuritis, the optic disc appears normal. The associated visual field defect is usually a centrocaecal scotoma.

49) c. The *p* value measures the probability that the null hypothesis is false.

50) b. Cardiff acuity cards are suitable for children between 1- to 2-year-old. Kay pictures are used for children with sufficient language skills

to name the pictures (usually age 2). Sheridan-Gardner test is usually used for children age 3 or older.

51) c. Stickler is the commonest aetiology for childhood retinal detachment. The associated systemic features include facial abnormality (Pierre Robin syndrome), arachnodactyly, joint hyperflexibility, deafness and mitral regurgitation.

52) b. Poor levator function ptosis (less than 4mm) requires brow suspension. Autologous fascia lata can be used but it is usually necessary to wait until the age of about 5 years for a child's leg to be sufficiently developed to harvest fascia lata. There is a variety of non-autogenous suspensory material which can be used, but all materials have the disadvantages of potential infection, extrusion, breakage, or foreign body granuloma formation.

53) c. Choroidal melanoma is a dense tumour with low blood flow and high absorption of ultrasound. This causes low reflectivity or acoustic hollowness. With brachy- or radiotherapy treatment, the reflectivity increases. A haemangioma has very high blood flow and low absorption of ultrasound, resulting in high reflectivity.

54) a. Or   -0.5DS/+1.00DC

55) d. The patient has right monofixation. The right eye is used to fixate distant objects. The same image falls within the suppressed area in left fovea. Both foveae are able to fixate near objects simultaneously.

56) a. This is the minimal thickness for LASIK. The amount of refractive error to be corrected also has a bearing. This question was asked in September 2010 exam paper.

57) b. This location is taken as the standard (default) reference plane because it corresponds to the centre of the papillomacular bundle of the RNFL. The visual acuity is usually preserved until the late stage in glaucoma therefore the papillomacular bundle (which serves the fovea) would be expected to have a stable thickness over time. However, there are other reference planes that have been proposed.

58) d. Long term steroid use causes hypokalaemia. Other systemic side-effects include peptic ulceration, Cushing syndrome, pancreatitis, hyperlipidaemia, psychological dependence and proximal myopathy.

59) a. This is also known as power of the test. An increase in power means less chance of committing a Type 2 error.

60) d. A similar question was asked in the September 2010 MCQ paper. Twenty percent of MS patients present with optic neuritis. The

overall 10-year risk of developing MS following an acute episode of optic neuritis is 38%. Even when brain lesions are detected on the MRI scan, clinical MS does not develop within 10 years in 44% of patients.

61) c. Thin retinal haemorrhage appears highly reflective however causes attenuation after more than 200µm deep and blocks the reflections from deeper layers.

62) a. The visual loss does not tend to improve with time and in a small percentage of patients can deteriorate further. The typical visual field defect is inferior altitudinal.

63) b. Sudan black stains lipid which is present in abundance in this tumour. SCC consists of squamous cells with prominent nuclei and abundant eosinophilic cytoplasm. BCC exhibit the pathognomonic palisading of cells at the periphery of the tumour. Merkel cell carcinoma arises from neuroendocrine tissue and shows cells with scarce cytoplasm with numerous mitotic figures.

64) d. BRVO can rarely cause rubeosis iridis, however retinal neovascularisation tends to occur before this.

65) a. FLAIR stands for fluid-attenuated inversion recovery, is employed for fluid suppression and provides good delineation for paraventricular pathology e.g. periventricular plaque in MS, acute infarct.

66) c. According to the GMC guidance, patient's information must not be disclosed to a third party such as a solicitor, police officer or officer of a court without the patient's express consent, unless it is required by law or can be justified in the public interest. Information must be disclosed if ordered to do so by a judge or presiding officer of a court. However, if the information appears to be irrelevant such as information about a patient's relative who is not involved in the proceedings, the doctor should object to the judge or the presiding officer order.

67) b. The visual acuity may be normal. Optic nerve hypoplasia is more common in children of diabetic mothers.

68) d. Exudative retinal detachment occurs in the absence of retinal breaks or traction. A retinoschisis can develop breaks in the inner and outer layers.

69) c. The choroidal phase usually occurs between 8 – 12 seconds after the fluorescein dye is injected. This time is dependent on various factors e.g. age, cardiovascular function, carotid stenosis etc.

Fluorescein pervades the plasma at the peripheral of the blood vessel. In fundal photograph, the plasma is difficult to visualise and only the axial blood column is visible.

70) b. In the EUCLID trial, lisinopril showed a significant reduction in the progression of diabetic retinopathy over 2 years.

71) c. Fungi are also stained with Calcoflour white. Giemsa stain is for Chlamydia.

72) d. Unilateral cataracts usually occurs sporadically affecting healthy infants. It is usually not associated with systemic disease. About two-thirds of congenital cataracts are bilateral. Not all bilateral cataracts are associated with systemic disorder.

73) b. The confidence interval is not given in the question. The null hypothesis is rejected (i.e. there is a statistical significant difference between the treated and no treatment group) if the confidence interval is set at 95% but not at 99%.

74) a. A combination of laboratory tests, clinical and histopathology findings are required to diagnose temporal arteritis. Diagnostic sensitivity increases to 97-99% with the combination of ESR and CRP. Histopathological findings persist for at least 2-6 weeks after the initiation of steroid.

75) c. The technique provides good anatomical information but limited functional or physiological data.

76) b. Pauciarticular arthritis is confined to four or fewer joints. The common complaint in a child affected with uveitis is poor vision. This can due to glaucoma, band keratopathy or macula oedema. Topical steroid treatment is usually sufficient.

77) d. Acetazolamide increases the bicarbonate excretion from the kidneys and can cause metabolic acidosis.

78) c. The wavefront aberrometer can detect various higher-order optical aberrations which can be subtracted individually from the patient's wavefront map. This allows the particular type of aberration that causes symptom to be identified.

79) a. von Kossa stains calcium black. Alizarin red can also be used, and calcium is stained red.

80) b. The GMC advises whenever possible that a doctor should not provide medical care to anyone whom has a close personal relationship.

81) c. The larger the p value, the more likely the null hypothesis is true.

82) a. Other organisms include *Staph. Epidermidis, Corynebacterium spp* or *Candida spp.*

83) a. If a patient has retinoblastoma and the parents are healthy, the risk to other siblings is 2%. The risk to the patient's offspring is 1%. If one of the patient's parents has retinoblastoma, the risk to other siblings is 40%. The risk of having an affected offspring is 4%.

84) c. Patients with cross-fixation usually have similar visual acuity in both eyes. Occlusion therapy is not indicated.

85) d. Pars planitis is a form of intermediate uveitis with snowbanking or snowball formations in the inferior part of the retina or vitreous. It affects children more frequently. The other complications associated with this condition include cystoids macular oedema, cataract, glaucoma, peripheral vasoproliferative tumour and ocular hypotension (which may lead to hypotonous maculopathy).

86) a. Epiphora occurs between 3 to 6% of newborns. Less than 10% of these occur bilaterally. Nasolacrimal duct dysfunction is common in craniofacial abnormalities.

87) c. Tropicamide is a muscarinic antagonist. It can precipitate angle closure and tachycardia. It can exacerbate ataxic dysarthria, cerebellar signs and increase the risk of seizure.

88) d. Dacryoscintigraphy should be performed for incomplete obstruction of the proximal canaliculus. The procedure involves instillation of a radionuclide tracer into the conjunctival sac. In dacryocystogram, the canaliculus is catheterised therefore dilating the partially obstructed proximal part of the canaliculus and prevent useful information to be obtained.

89) d. Chronic anterior uveitis can cause raised IOP in children with JIA. The intracranial pressure is raised in IIH however, the ocular venous return should remain normal.

90) c. For babies born before 27 weeks gestational age (i.e. up to 26 weeks and 6 days), the first ROP screening examination should be undertaken at 30 to 31 weeks postmenstrual age. Babies born between 27 and 32 weeks gestational age (i.e. up to 31 weeks and 6 days) should be screened between 4 to 5 weeks postnatal age. Babies born >32 weeks gestational age but with birthweight <1501 grams, should be screened between 4 to 5 weeks postnatal age.

EMQ Paper 2

A) Eales disease

B) Vitreous haemorrhage secondary to PVD

C) Retinal artery macroaneurysm

D) Proliferative sickle-cell retinopathy

E) Proliferative diabetic retinopathy

F) Hypertensive retinopathy

G) Idiopathic polypoidal choroidal vasculopathy

H) Central retinal vein occlusion

I) Ocular ischaemic syndrome

J) Familial exudative vitreoretinopathy

Select the most likely diagnosis for each patient.

1) A 30-year-old healthy African man presents with recurrent vitreous haemorrhage. Dilated fundoscopy reveals peripheral retinal haemorrhage and vascular sheathing in the superotemporal quadrant. New vessels are evident in the same area. The fellow eye is normal.

2) A 72-year-old complains of left blurry vision. He is diabetic and hypertensive. There are corneal oedema, episcleral injection, and optic disc neovascularisation in the left eye. The retinal arteries are pulsatile. The fellow eye has scattered dot haemorrahages and no vascular changes.

A) -1.00D

B) 0.00D

C) +1.00D

D) +1.50D

E) +2.00D

F) +2.50D

G) +3.50D

H) +4.50D

I) +5.50D

J) +6.50D

A patient needs +2.00D to see distance clearly and can tolerate up to +3.50D without getting blurred. His cycloplegic refraction is +4.50DS.

3) What is the absolute hypermetropia?

4) What is the facultative hypermetropia?

A) Transpupillary diode laser therapy within 48 hours
B) Cryotherapy within 48 hours
C) Argon laser within 48 hours
D) Vitrectomy within 48 hours
E) Continue to monitor daily
F) Examine 3-5 days post treatment and weekly for signs of regression
G) Examine 5-7 days post treatment and weekly for signs of regression
H) Examine 8-12 days post treatment and fortnightly for signs of regression
I) Arrange for retreatment 10-14 days after the first treatment
J) Discharge patient

For each question, choose the recommended action based on the UK Retinopathy of Prematurity Guideline 2008.

5) A baby born at 26 weeks of gestation was found to have stage 3 ROP with plus disease in zone 1 at screening.

6) A baby just had ROP treatment in theatre.

A) Dominant optic neuropathy of Kjer
B) Diabetic papillopathy
C) Leber hereditary optic neuropathy
D) Spheno-orbital meningioma
E) Posterior ischaemic optic neuropathy
F) Nutritional optic neuropathy
G) Demyelinating disease
H) Wolfram syndrome
I) Friedreich ataxia
J) Non-organic visual loss

Select the most likely diagnosis for each patient.

7) A 25-year-old presents with painless, rapid monocular visual loss. His acuity is 6/36 in the affected eye. There are peripapillary telangiectasia and a dense centrocecal scotoma. The temporal region of the optic disc is swollen but there is no leak on the FFA.

8) A vagrant was admitted with confusion, peripheral neuropathy and abdominal pain two days ago. He now complains of painless bilateral poor vision. Fundoscopy is normal.

A) Physostigmine
B) Ecothiopate
C) Pyridostigmine
D) Cannabis
E) Diazepam
F) Pilocarpine 0.1%
G) Pilocarpine 1%
H) Cocaine 4%
I) Hydroxyamphetamine 1%
J) Adrenaline 1:1000

Select the most appropriate drug for each description.

9) Treatment for myasthenia gravis.

10) Dilates a Horner pupil with postganglionic lesion.

A) Capillary haemangioma
B) Cavernous haemangioma
C) Lymphangioma
D) Carotid-cavernous fistula
E) Primary orbital varices
F) Ruptured dermoid cyst
G) Acute dacryoadenitis
H) Malignant pleomorphic adenocarcinoma
I) Preseptal orbital cellulitis
J) Orbital cellulitis

Select the most likely diagnosis for each patient.

11) A 6-year-old presents with a painless, bluish mass on the nasal quadrant of the upper lid. The lesion enlarges whenever he coughs.

12) A 10-year-old presents with an acute red, painful swelling on the lateral part of the upper lid. There is a downward and inward dystopia. The conjunctiva is inflamed at the upper lateral quadrant.

A) *Staphylococcus aureus*
B) *Staphylococcus epidermidis*
C) *Streptococcus pneumonia*
D) *Haemophilus influenza*
E) Human papilloma virus
F) Herpes simplex virus
G) Herpes zoster virus
H) Poxvirus
I) Adenovirus
J) Togavirus

Select the likely pathogen causing each lesion.

13) Multiple pale, waxy and umbilicated nodules.

14) Erythematous macular lesion on the face which develops into thin-walled cysts and surrounded by yellow crust.

A) Oc.aciclovir 5 times daily
B) G.dexamethasone 0.1% qds and g.cyclopentolate 1% tds
C) Oc.aciclovir 5 times daily and g.dexamethasone 0.1% qds
D) Oc.aciclovir tds, g.dexamethasone 0.1% qds, g.cyclopentolate 1% tds
E) G.dexamethasone 0.1% two hourly and aciclovir tablet 400mg bd
F) Aciclovir tablet 400mg 5 times daily, g.dexamethasone 0.1% qds and g.cyclopentolate 1% tds
G) Aciclovir tablet 800mg 5 times daily
H) Aciclovir tablet 800mg 5 times daily, g.dexamethasone 0.1% qds and g.cyclopentolate 1% tds
I) g.dexamethasone 0.1% qds and g.chloramphenicol qds
J) g.chloramphenicol qds

Select the most appropriate treatment for each presentation.

15) A 68-year-old presents with a hazy corneal stroma temporally and 1+ cell in the anterior chamber. There is deep corneal vascularisation at the same site. The cornea is not stained with fluorescein. He complains his eye had never been the same since an ulcer a few years ago.

16) A 70-year-old with left hemifrontal (obeying the midline) scabs and vesicles presents with blurry left vision. There is poor staining of fine, branching defects on the cornea epithelium. The eye is quiet.

A) High corneal astigmatism
B) Previous refractive surgery
C) IOP of 30mmHg
D) Patient on tamsulosin
E) Fuchs endothelial guttata
F) Posterior pole cataract
G) BP 195/95
H) Diabetic with blood sugar level of 12mmol
I) Myopia of -6.00D
J) Previous vitrectomy

Select the most likely aetiology for each complication.

17) Persistent postoperative corneal oedema.

18) Intraoperative suprachoroidal haemorrhage.

A) Steroid induced raised intraocular pressure
B) Epithelial downgrowth
C) Phacoanaphylactic uveitis
D) Fuchs heterochromic cyclitis
E) Pigment dispersion syndrome
F) Plateau iris syndrome
G) Pseudoexfoliation syndrome
H) Iridocorneal endothelial syndrome
I) Posner-Schlossman syndrome
J) Toxic anterior segment syndrome

Select the most likely diagnosis for each patient.

19) A 31-year-old complains of intermittent blurry vision his right eye every time he plays squash. Examination reveals partial loss of iris pupillary ruff and mid-periphery iris transillumination defect in the both eyes. The IOP is normal.

20) A patient had a complicated cataract operation 6 months ago. He presents with painful blurry vision. There is sectoral corneal oedema with an underlying gray membrane on the cornea endothelial surface. The pupil is distorted. There are 2+ cells in the anterior chamber. The IOP is 38mmHg.

A) Observation every 3 months
B) Transpupillary thermotherapy
C) Argon laser photocoagulation
D) Brachytherapy with ruthenium-106
E) Brachytherapy with iodine-125
F) Charged particle irradiation
G) Transcleral choroidectomy
H) Enucleation
I) Exenteration
J) Systemic chemotherapy

Select the most appropriate treatment for the intraocular lesion.

21) A 41-year-old presents with a temporal choroidal mass associated with exudative retinal detachment. His visual acuity is 6/9. Ultrasound measures the lesion height at 7mm and base diameter at 12mm.

22) A 58-year-old presents with shallow anterior chamber, rubeosis iridis and a choroidal lesion in his left eye. His acuities are perception of light in the left eye and 6/6 right. There is exudative retinal detachment. The mass is 14mm in height and has a 22mm base diameter. MRI orbit shows no extraocular involvement and the liver function test is normal.

A) Barrier laser
B) Pars plana vitrectomy, barrier laser and gas tamponade
C) Pars plana vitrectomy and cryotherapy
D) Pars plana vitrectomy, retinotomy and silicone oil
E) Pars plana vitrectomy, retinotomy and 360^0 scleral buckle
F) Full thickness scleral decompression and drainage
G) Full thickness scleral decompression, drainage and 360^0 cryotherapy
H) 360^0 scleral buckle and cryotherapy
I) Pneumatic retinopexy
J) Observation

Choose the most appropriate intervention for the clinical scenario.

23) A patient presents with optic disc pit and adjacent retinal detachment. The patient is asymptomatic and the visual acuity is 6/6.

24) A 50-year-old man presents with 360^0 peripheral choroidal effusion in one eye. There is no past ophthalmic history. There is no tobacco dusting and the IOP is 20mmHg.

A) Posterior scleritis
B) Sympathetic ophthalmia
C) Uveal effusion syndrome
D) Choroidal melanoma
E) Vogt-Koyanagi-Harada syndrome
F) Metastasis to the choroid
G) Sarcoidosis
H) Tuberculosis
I) Multifocal choroiditis with panuveitis
J) Birdshot chorioretinopathy

Select the most likely diagnosis for each patient.

25) A 34-year-old presents with optic disc oedema and multiple serous retinal detachments in one eye. The fellow eye has diffused choroidal infiltrates. The patient also complains of hearing loss. There is no history of ocular trauma or surgery.

26) An Indian gentleman complains of poor vision. He has cells in both anterior chambers. Fundoscopy reveals perivenous exudates and sheathing. There are multiple deep yellow lesions in the fundi and discrete preretinal small lesions inferiorly.

A) Knapp procedure
B) Inverse Knapp procedure
C) Hummelsheim procedure
D) Base-up prism
E) Base-down prism
F) Harada-Ito procedure
G) Faden procedure
H) Superior rectus recession and inferior rectus resection
I) Botulinum toxin to the medial rectus
J) Maximum medial rectus resection and lateral rectus recession

Select the most appropriate management for each patient.

27) A 60-year-old with unilateral total sixth nerve palsy for more than a year.

28) A 4-year-old has limited upgaze across the horizontal plane in the left eye. The right eye has full range of movement. There is chin lift.

A) Chalazion
B) Squamous cell papilloma
C) Basal cell papilloma
D) Eccrine hidrocystoma
E) Keratoacanthoma
F) Epidermoid cyst
G) Neurofibroma
H) Xanthelasma
I) Pilomatricoma
J) Pyogenic granuloma

Select the most appropriate diagnosis based on the histological reports.

29) The microscopic examination reveals a keratin-filled cavity within the dermis lined by keratinised stratified squamous epithelium.

30) The lesion shows proliferation of Schwann cells and fibroblast.

A) Acoustic neuroma
B) Nasapharyngeal tumour
C) High-flow carotid-cavernous fistula
D) Low-flow carotid-cavernous fistula
E) Cavernous sinus thrombosis
F) Invasive pituitary adenoma
G) Unruptured intracavernous carotid aneurysm
H) Optic nerve sheath meningioma
I) Tolosa-Hunt syndrome
J) Thyroid ophthalmopathy

Choose the most likely diagnosis for each patient.

31) A 50-year-old Chinese man presents with distant binocular diplopia. There is a right face turn. The right eye is slightly proptosed. He also has been experiencing frequent right nasal obstruction and epistaxis. There is no hearing loss or corneal anaesthesia.

32) A 45-year-old lady complains of worsening binocular diplopia over the last 2 months. There are limited movement of the left eye in up, down, medial and lateral gazes. The left pupil is smaller and there is a mild ptosis on the same side. There is no ocular pain, conjunctival hyperaemia or proptosis.

A) Classical angina
B) Variant angina
C) Unstable angina
D) Pulmonary embolism
E) Musculoskeletal chest pain
F) Anaphylactic shock
G) Diabetic ketoacidosis
H) Hyperglycaemic hyperosmolar non-ketotic acidosis
I)   Status epilepticus
J)   Acute asthma attack

Select the most likely diagnosis for the emergency situation mentioned.

33) A 65-year-old lady complains of sudden onset gripping, central chest pain to the out-patient nurse in the waiting room. She takes her glyceryl trinitrate spray which seems to relieve the symptom. The ECG reveals depressed ST and T wave inversion.

34) A diabetic patient complains of difficulty in breathing and feeling nauseous. She just had eye photograph taken with strong flashes. Her skin has an orange tinge discolouration. She has very warm peripheries and a bounding pulse. Her face is swollen. The blood pressure is 80/40mmHg and heart rate 160beats/min.

A) Pellucid marginal degeneration
B) Terrien marginal degeneration
C) Keratoconus
D) Fuchs endothelial dystrophy
E) Lattice dystrophy
F) Granular dystrophy
G) Macular dystrophy
H) Thiel-Behnke dystrophy
I)   Meesman dystrophy
J)   Spheroidal degeneration

Choose the most likely diagnosis from the corneal histological findings.

35) There is central stromal thinning and patchy loss of Bowman layer associated with oedema of the adjacent epithelial cells.

36) The stromal deposits on the cornea show green birefringence when viewed with polarised light. The endothelial layer appears to be normal.

A) Macular grid laser
B) Focal laser
C) Intravitreal triamcinolone injection
D) Intravitreal bevacizumab injection
E) Intravitreal tissue plasminogen activator injection
F) Panretinal photocoagulation
G) YAG vitreolysis
H) Vitrectomy
I) Observe 3-monthly
J) FFA to assess macular ischaemia

Select the most appropriate management for the conditions below.

37) A lady with diabetes and ocular hypertension had 4 sittings of macular grid laser to both eyes over a year. Her HbA$_{1C}$ is 7.2%. Her visual acuities are 6/12. The OCT scan reveals diffuse macula oedema.

38) A 33-year-old poorly controlled diabetic has not been attending his follow-up appointments. He presents with a dense premacular subhyaloid haemorrhage. There is vitreous and wide spread dot blot haemorrhages.

A) Third nerve nucleus centre
B) Midbrain area adjacent to the red nucleus
C) Rostral lower midbrain
D) Rostral upper pontine
E) Junction of the posterior cerebral and superior cerebellar arteries
F) Posterior communicating artery adjacent to the third nerve
G) Cavernous sinus
H) Orbital apex
I) Superior orbital area
J) Inferior orbital area

Select the most likely site of the lesion involved in each case.

39) A 45-year-old presents with gradual onset of diplopia. Examination reveals limited right eye movement on adduction, downgaze and upgaze. The right pupil is mid-dilated. There is mild right proptosis, inferior dystopia and reduced sensation of the forehead. The fellow eye is normal.

40) A 70-year-old had a fall in a month ago. She complains of hearing bruit in her head and diplopia. Examination reveals uniocular limited eye movement with bilateral conjunctival hyperaemia and proptosis.

There are only 8 options in this question.

A) Acetazolamide tablets
B) Bimatoprost
C) Brinzolamide
D) Brimonidine
E) Pilocarpine
F) Propine
G) Tafluprost
H) Timolol

Select the appropriate anti-glaucoma treatment for each scenario.

41) A 66-year-old gentleman presents with moderate corneal oedema, mild anterior chamber inflammation and IOP of 30mmHg. Four months ago, he was treated for herpes zoster ophthalmicus. He is on amitryptyline for trigeminal neuralgia.

42) A 70-year-old lady had her topical medication for glaucoma changed recently. Her intraocular pressure is controlled now. She mentions her droopy lids have improved with the treatment.

A) Hughes tarso-conjunctival flap and skin graft
B) Posterior lamellar graft and Fricke flap ⟵skin muscle.
C) Tenzel semicircular flap
D) Direct closure with lateral cantholysis
E) Lateral periosteal flap and skin
F) Mustarde cheek rotation flap (vertical deep, NOT horizontal).
G) Glabellar flap
H) Sliding tarsoconjunctival flap and skin mobilisation
I) Cutler-Beard lower lid bridge flap
J) Full thickness tarsoconjunctival skin graft from the fellow upper lid.

Select the most suitable surgical technique for the eyelid defects.

43) The surgeon has just excised the left lower lid lesion with the appropriate margin. The horizontal lid defect is about 80% and vertical defect 1cm. The left visual acuity is 6/9 and the right eye has advanced age related macular degeneration.

44) A Moh's micrographic surgery has removed the lateral half of the upper lid and lateral canthal tendons.

A) Linear IgA disease
B) Mucous membrane pemphigoid
C) Stevens-Johnson syndrome
D) Toxic epidermal necrolysis _Multiorgan failure t rep wi._
E) Epidermolysis bullosa
F) Bullous impetigo
G) Staphyloccal folliculitis
H) Bullous pemphigoid
I) Bacteraemia
J) Septic shock

Choose the most likely diagnosis for the clinical scenario.

45) A 10-year-old has been referred by the paediatrician. He has multiple clusters of blister on his hands, feet and face only. The onset was abrupt and no triggers were found. Examination reveals bilateral symblepharon, corneal epithelial defect and vascularisation.

46) A 30-year-old was treated 10 days ago with trimethoprim for a urinary tract infection. She presents to the A&E with watery eyes and acute blistering of her skin. She has target lesions and inflamed mucosa in her mouth and throat. There is severe bilateral conjunctivitis and pseudomembrane. She is apyrexial and haemodynamically stable.

A) ACCORD
B) ADVANCE
C) BOLT
D) CARDS
E) DIRECT
F) EUCLID
G) FIELD
H) HOPE
I) RASS
J) UKPDS

Select the clinical trial which corresponds to each statement. _T2DM_

47) Fenofibrate with simvastatin reduces the odds of diabetic retinopathy progression by 40% compared to simvastatin alone over 4 years.

48) Over a period of 5 years, candesartan resulted in 34% regression of _T2DM_ retinopathy in type II diabetes.

A) Vitamin A
B) Vitamin B_1
C) Vitamin B_6
D) Vitamin B_{12}
E) Vitamin C
F) Vitamin D
G) Vitamin E
H) Vitamin K
I) Selenium
J) Zinc and copper

Select the most appropriate treatment for the conditions mentioned.

49) Pernicious anaemia related optic neuropathy

50) Xerophthalmia

A) Panretinal photocoagulation
B) Macular grid laser
C) Intense topical steroid and oral acetazolamide
D) Posterior subtenon triamcinolone
E) Oral acetazolamide and oral steroid
F) Intravitreal triamcinolone
G) Intravitreal ganciclovir
H) Intravenous ganciclovir
I) Intravenous aciclovir
J) Intravenous methylprednisolone

Select the most appropriate treatment for each patient.

51) A 35-year-old Ethiopian lady presents with severe visual blurring in both eyes. She has been feeling unwell for the past weeks. Fundoscopy reveals confluent yellow-white areas with associated flame shaped haemorrhages in both eyes. There is perivascular sheathing. Her CD4+ count is 45cells/µl.

52) A 30-year-old with a history of multiple sclerosis is seen in a routine follow-up clinic. She complains her vision is getting worse in the left eye. Her acuities are 6/6 in the right eye and 6/12 in the left. She has flare in the anterior chamber and moderate vitritis. There is left cystoids macular oedema.

A) Acute posterior multifocal placoid pigment epitheliopathy
B) Birdshot retinochoroidopathy
C) Punctuate inner choroidopathy
D) Presumed ocular histoplasmosis syndrome
E) Fundus flavimaculatus
F) Stargardt disease
G) Best disease
H) Familial dominant drusen
I) Sorsby pseudo-inflammatory dystrophy
J) Juvenile retinoschisis

Choose the most likely diagnosis based on the FFA findings.

53) There are multiple areas of hypofluorescence in the mid-periphery retina in the venous phase. These lesions and the optic disc hyperfluoresced four minutes later.

54) There is absence of choroidal fluorescence in arteriovenous phase and hyperfluorescence at centre of the macula in the late phase.

A) Posner-Schlossman syndrome
B) Fuchs heterochromic cyclitis
C) Chronic angle closure glaucoma
D) Primary open angle glaucoma
E) Pigment dispersion syndrome
F) Aqueous misdirection syndrome
G) Plateau iris syndrome
H) Schwartz-Mazuo syndrome
I) Alport syndrome
J) Iridocorneal endothelial syndrome

Select the most likely diagnosis for each patient.

55) A high myope presents with blurry vision and photopsia. The cornea is oedematous and the IOP is 45mmHg. Gonioscopy shows opened angle. Fundoscopy reveals multiple retinal tears and a retinal detachment.

56) A deaf 18-year-old was referred by his renal physician after complaining of poor vision. Band-like defects and multiple vesicles can be seen in the deep corneal layers. Pigment dusting, corectopia, ectropion uveau and iris atrophy are also seen. The IOP's are in the mid-thirties. There is asymmetrical optic disc cupping.

A) Thayer-Martin medium

B) Lowerstein- Jensen medium

C) Blood agar

D) Chocolate agar

E) Cooked meat broth agar

F) Non-nutrient agar laden with *E.coli*

G) Sabouraud agar

H) Thioglycate agar

I) MacConkey agar

J) McCoy agar

Select the most appropriate investigative medium for each microorganism.

57) *Neisseria gonorrhea*

58) *Chlamydia trachomatis*

A) Bulbar palsy

B) Pseudobulbar palsy

C) Syringobulbia

D) Wallenberg syndrome

E) Nothangel syndrome

F) Parinaud syndrome

G) Balint syndrome

H) Steele-Richarson-Olszewski syndrome

I) Chronic progressive external ophthalmoplegia

J) Oculogyric crisis

Choose the most likely diagnosis for each description.

59) A 60-year-old presents to A&E with acute unsteadiness, double vision, left-sided facial pain and hoarseness. He has a wide-based gait and intentional tremor. There is a mild left ptosis, and a fast phase nystagmus towards the left.

60) A middle age man complains of difficulty in reading and looking up. Examination reveals defective near convergence and limited upgaze. There is skew deviation. Lid retraction occurs during attempted upgaze but disappear in downgaze. There is light-near dissociation of the pupils.

A) Aicardi syndrome
B) Allagille syndrome *posterior embryotoxon*
C) CHARGE syndrome
D) Congenital rubella
E) Cornelia de Lange syndrome
F) De Morsier syndrome
G) Down syndrome
H) Fabry disease
I) Hallerman-Streiff syndrome *membranous cataract.*
J) Lowe syndrome

galactosemia - reducing substance urine.
Lowe - amino acid
Fabry's - sediments.
Wilson - copper
Alport's - blood.

Select the likely diagnosis for each clinical scenario.

61) A 4-year-old has left esotropia intermittently. The boy has a beak-shaped nose, micrognathia and hypotrichosis. There is premature dentine eruption and enamel hypoplasia. There is bilateral microphthalmos and membranous white cataract. He is very short for his age.

62) A toddler has been under the care of the paediatrician since aminoaciduria was detected. Both his uncles had cataract removal at a young age. The child has mental developmental delay, hypotonia and abnormal skull shape. He has lamellar cataract in both eyes.

A) Wound leak
B) Ciliary body shutdown
C) Choroidal detachment
D) Suprachoroidal haemorrhage
E) Pupillary block
F) Aqueous misdirection syndrome
G) Overfiltration
H) Uveitic glaucoma
I)   Steroid induced glaucoma
J) Sclerostomy block

Select the most likely cause for each situation.

63) Two days post-trabeculectomy, the anterior chamber is shallow and the IOP is 6mmHg. The bleb is flat and Seidel test is negative. Fundoscopy is unremarkable.

64) Two days post-trabeculectomy, the anterior chamber is shallow and the IOP is 30mmHg. The bleb is flat and Seidel test is negative. The peripheral iridotomy is patent. Fundoscopy is unremarkable.

A) Doppler carotid ultrasound
B) Doppler temporal artery ultrasound
C) OCT
D) Ocular B-scan
E) CT head
F) MRI T1 weighted
G) MRI T2 weighted
H) MR angiography
I) Skull X-ray
J) FFA

Select the most useful investigation for each patient.

65) A 70-year-old diabetic complains of left blurry vision. There are left corneal oedema, anterior chamber cell and conjunctival injection. The left pupil is mid-dilated and reacts poorly to light. Fundoscopy reveals tortuous and dilated retinal veins. The ESR and CRP are normal.

66) A 13-year-old accidentally shot his eye while playing with a ball bearing gun. The iris and vitreous are prolapsed through the temporal corneal limbus.

A) Retinal tear at 12 o'clock
B) Retinal tear at 4 o'clock
C) Retinal tear at 6 o'clock
D) Retinal tear at 8 o'clock
E) Retinal tear at 10 o'clock
F) Superior temporal retinoschitic tear
G) Inferior giant tear
H) Superior retinal dialysis
I) Macular hole
J) Inferior equatorial tear

Locate the position of the retinal defect for each retinal detachment.

67) Bullous inferior retinal detachment with the macular and superior retina attached

68) The entire superior retina is detached and undulated during ocular movement. An inferior retina wedge is attached between 4 to 6 clock hours.

A) Treat the right eye first and the left a fortnight later with intravitreal ranibizumab
B) Treat the left eye first and the right a fortnight later with intravitreal ranibizumab
C) Treat the right eye first and the left a month later with intravitreal ranibizumab
D) Treat the right eye first and the left a month later with intravitreal ranibizumab
E) Treat both eyes simultaneously with intravitreal ranibizumab
F) Withhold intravitreal ranibizumab until an indocyanine green angiogram is performed to assess the whole lesion
G) Withhold intravitreal ranibizumab until the IOP is reduced to 25mmHg with topical anti-glaucoma treatment
H) Treat with intravitreal ranibizumab and perform an anterior chamber paracentesis to reduce the IOP at the same sitting
I) Treat with intravitreal ranibizumab and give a post-procedure course of oral acetazolamide
J) The patient is not suitable for intravitreal ranibizumab treatment

Based on the Royal College of Ophthalmologists guideline for age-related macular degeneration management, select the recommended treatment.

69) A 67-year-old has been referred for bilateral distorted visions. Her right visual acuity is 6/18, and left 6/36. Fundoscopy reveals bilateral drusen and subfoveal lesions. The FFA shows classic choroidal neovascular membrane in both eyes.

70) A 70-year-old patient has foveal haemorrhage which constitutes more than 50% of the total choroidal neovascular membrane on the FFA. The acuity is 6/60 and IOP 35mmHg.

A) Non-refractive convergence excess
B) Near esotropia
C) Early onset esotropia
D) Distance esotropia
E) Fully accommodative esotropia
F) Partially accommodative esotropia
G) Paretic esotropia
H) Consecutive esotropia
I) Convergence spasm
J) Cyclical esotropia

Select the most likely type of strabismus for each orthoptic finding.

71) An 18-month-old with the findings below.

   Visual acuity: 6/9 both eyes

   Cover test: alternating/left convergent squint

   Prism cover test for near and distant: BO 40PD

   Ocular movement: comitant deviation, with up-shoot of the left
   eye on dextroversion

   Refraction: +2.0D both eyes

72) A 7-year-old has the following orthoptic findings.

   Visual acuity: 6/6 both eyes

   Cover test: right esotropia

   Prism cover test: BO 10PD for near; BO 40PD for distant

   Ocular movement: incomitant deviation

   Refraction: RE +0.5D   LE +0.75D

A) Embryonal sarcoma
B) Lymphoproliferative tumour
C) Metastatic carcinoma to the optic nerve
D) Optic nerve glioma
E) Optic nerve sheath meningioma
F) Neuroblastoma
G) Orbital cellulitis
H) Spontaneous orbital haemorrhage
I) Lacrimal gland tumour
J) Thyroid orbitopathy

Select the most likely diagnosis for each patient.

73) A 6-year-old girl develops a slow-onset and painless left visual loss. There is mild axial proptosis. The optic nerve is swollen and there is wide spread flame-shaped retinal haemorrhages. CT scan shows fusiform enlargement of the optic nerve and a wide optic canal.

74) A five-year-old presents with non-traumatic periocular ecchymosis, subconjunctival haemorrhage and proptosis. The CT scan shows a mass inside the lateral orbital wall. There is no bone erosion.

A) Amoxicillin
B) Erythromycin
C) Cefuroxime
D) Moxifloxacin
E) Metronidazole
F) Trimethoprim
G) Tamsulosin hydrochloride
H) Bethanechol chloride
I) Duloxetine
J) Oxybutynin hydrochloride

Select the most likely drug for each description.

75) Prescribing this medication is likely to increase the risk of myopathy in patients on simvastatin.

76) Patients taking this treatment for urinary problem may have an increase risk of complication during cataract operation.

A) Urgent IV methylprednisolone
B) Urgent lateral canthotomy
C) Urgent IV acetazolomide
D) Urgent medial orbital wall repair
E) Medial orbital wall repair between 2 -3 weeks
F) Oral antibiotic and high dose oral steroid
G) Refer to the orbital specialist soon
H) Suture the skin laceration
I) Subtenon triamcinolone
J) No immediate intervention and review a few days

Select the most appropriate management for each clinical scenario.

77) A 45-year-old man was punched in the right eye. The vision has been deteriorating rapidly while waiting to be seen. There is severe chemosis and lid oedema. The IOP is 70mmHg. Fundoscopy reveals spontaneous arterial pulsation. The eye movement is severely restricted.

78) A 22-year-old has been involved in a fight. He complains of diplopia. There is lid swelling, subconjunctival haemorrhage and a 1cm laceration 2cm below the lid margin. The eye is quiet. Fundoscopy shows commotio retinae inferior to the macula. CT scan reveals medial orbital wall fracture with swollen orbital tissue. There is no medial rectus entrapment.

There are only 9 options available in this question.

A) Kearns-Sayre syndrome
B) Oculopharyngeal dystrophy
C) Thyroid ophthalmopathy
D) Myotonic dystrophy
E) Myasthenia gravis
F) Orbital pseudotumour
G) Internuclear ophthalmoplegia
H) Third nerve palsy
I) Excessive tiredness

Must
- Progressive external ophthalmoplegia
- < 20 years
- pigmentary retinal changes
+
1 of
- cerebellar dysfunction
- cardiac conduction defects
- CSF protein >100

Select the most likely diagnosis for each patient.

79) A teenager complains of worsening vision in the dark, bilateral ptosis and diplopia. He has been feeling lethargic and unsteady on his feet.

80) A patient complains of intermittent vertical diplopia and asymmetrical ptosis. Her symptoms usually improve with a short nap.

A) Amyloidosis
B) Ehlers-Danlos syndrome
C) Groenblad-Strandberg syndrome (Pseudoxanthoma)
D) Marfan syndrome
E) Paget disease
F) Sarcoidosis
G) Sturge-Weber syndrome
H) Tuberous sclerosis
I) Von Hippel-Lindau syndrome
J) Von Recklinghausen disease

Select the most likely diagnosis for each patient.

81) A patient has dark brown lines radiating from the optic discs toward the peripheral retinae. There is an associated area of retinal haemorrhage along one of the defects. There is 'plucked chicken' appearance of the skin on the neck and antecubital fossae.

82) A teenager has a bright yellow mulberry-like lesion in each fundus. He has red papules across his mid face. There are hypopigmented macules and firm, flesh-colour plaques on his truck. He is under the care of the neurologist for epilepsy and has periodic head scan.

A) A good randomised controlled trial applicable to target population
B) A systemic review of good quality case-control studies
C) A well conducted cohort study with low risk of bias directly applicable to target population
D) A case-control study with no confounding factors directly applicable to target population
E) A multicentre study with a common protocol
F) Case series
G) Case report
H) Cross-sectional study
I) Survey
J) Experts' consensus

Select the most appropriate type of study for each description.

83) To evaluate the outcome of an eye disease which occur 1 in 800,000 people.

84) Grade B strength of evidence (graded from A to D).

A) Behcet disease
B) Coat disease
C) Juvenile idiopathic arthritis
D) Leukaemia
E) Persistent hyperplastic primary vitreous
F) Retinoblastoma
G) Retinopathy of prematurity
H) Toxocariasis
I) Toxoplasmosis
J) Stickler syndrome

Choose the most likely condition for each patient.

85) A 7-year-old girl presents with rapid onset of left blurry vision. Examination reveals a left hypopyon. An inferior retinal granuloma with pars planitis is visible on indirect ophthalmoscopy. The right eye is normal. There is no significant past medical or ophthalmic history.

86) An 8-year-old boy complains of poor left vision. Indirect ophthalmoscopy shows a large area of retinal telangiectasia in the superotemporal quadrant. There is massive intraretinal exudate in the same area extending to the macula. The fellow eye is normal.

A) Haidinger's brush
B) Moore's lighting streak
C) Phosphene
D) Fortification spectrum
E) Purkinje phenomenon
F) Palinopsia
G) Pulfrich phenomenon
H) Polyopia
I) Riddoch phenomenon
J) Metamorphopsia

Select the most likely visual phenomenon for each case.

87) The patient complains of seeing a visual defect before experiencing a unilateral throbbing headache.

88) The patient is only aware of moving objects in the blind field and stationary ones are not seen.

A) Alstrom syndrome
B) Bardet-Biedl syndrome
C) Bassen-Kornzweig syndrome
D) Cockaryne syndrome
E) Leber congenital amaurosis
F) Hurler syndrome
G) Hunter syndrome
H) Kearn-Sayre syndrome
I) Refsum syndrome
J) Usher syndrome

Choose the most likely diagnosis associated with the pigmentary retinopathy patients.

89) The patient had an addition finger removed when she was a child. All her fingers are stubby. She is obese and has type 1 diabetes and renal dysfunction. There is bull's eye maculopathy.

90) A teenager has sensorimotor polyneuropathy and ichthyosis. He has cerebellar ataxia and cardiomyopathy. There is raised serum phytanic acid.

EMQ Paper 2 Answers

1. A. Despite the condition was first described by Henry Eales, a British ophthalmologist in the 19th century, this condition is rare in developed country nowadays and more common in the Indian subcontinent. The disease is recognised as primary vasculitis of unknown aetiology despite an association with tuberculosis has been proposed. The diagnostic feature of Eales disease is the peripheral venous inflammation which causes various degree of venous insufficiency. Bilaterality occurs in 50-90% of patients. Sickle cell retinopathy is a result of peripheral arterial occlusion.

2. I. The unilaterality of the findings is suggestive of ocular ischaemic syndrome. The condition is rare, and usually results from chronic hypoperfusion secondary to ipsilateral atherosclerotic carotid stenosis. The predisposing risk factors in this patient are diabetes, hypertension and his age. Spontaneous arterial pulsation is a common finding.

3. E. +2.00D. Absolute hypermetropia is the least amount of plus lenses needed for clear vision without cycloplegia. Manifest hypermetropia (+3.50D) is defined as the most plus correction that can be tolerated without blurring of vision and without cylcoplegia.

4. D. +1.50D. Facultative hypermetropia is the difference between absolute and manifest hypermetropia. Latent hypermetropia (+ 1.00D) is the difference between manifest hypermetropia and hypermetropia measured with cycloplegia.

5. A. This is classified as aggressive ROP and the current recommendation is for treatment within 48 hours. Transpupillary diode laser therapy is recommended over cryotherapy and argon laser, unless there is no access to the former. There are fewer incidences of epithelial cornea oedema, corneal burn and cataract formation with transpupillary diode laser.

6. G. Regression usually occurs at a mean of 5 days (range 2-14 days) after diode laser. Inflammation is likely to occur after treatment but usually have reduced by 5-7 days after. An examination at this stage is suitable to assess ROP regression.

7. C. The diagnostic features for this condition are the peripapillary telangiectasia and pseudoedema of the optic disc. Evidence of intraocular inflammation, extraocular neurological signs or periorbital pain should raise the question of an alternate diagnosis.

8. F. This patient is likely to have vitamin B deficiency. The condition presents with glove-and-stocking numbness and paraesthesia, cognitive decline, gastrointestinal symptoms and glossitis. Acutely, the optic discs may appear to be normal or hyperaemic. Over time, if untreated, permanent visual loss ensues and temporal pallor develops. Diffuse pallor is unusual.

9. C. This is an anticholinesterase. Despite careful titration of the dosage to maximally tolerated dose, ocular symptoms are frequently poorly controlled by this alone. Immunosuppressive drug is usually required.

10. J. In a postganglionic lesion, monoamine oxidase is not produced by the presynaptic neuron. The pupil dilates because the adrenaline is not broken down and the dilator pupillae muscle is denervation hypersensitive to adrenaline.

11. C. Lymphagioma usually presents in childhood and can present as anterior or posterior lesions. In this patient, the lesion is anterior as evident by the bluish lesion (venous blood) and a visible size increase with Valsalva manoeuvre. Posterior lesions have different signs – slowly progressive proptosis which may enlarge suddenly secondary to spontaneous bleed. The lesion can regress spontaneously, however urgent surgical attention is required for intralesional haemorrhage. Primary orbital varices do not have any external eye signs unless accentuated by Valsalva manoeuvre.

12. G. Another condition which commonly presents in childhood. Preseptal cellulitis is unlikely to cause dystopia, and ruptured dermoid cyst is not related with conjunctiva injection. Malignant adenocarcinoma may cause a similar picture but the presentation is not acute.

13. H. This is molluscum contagiosum.

14. A. Impetigo is a superficial skin infection caused by *Staph. aureus* or *Strep. pyogenes*.

15. F. The evaluation of keratouveitic treatment in the Herpetic Eye Disease Study 1was not completed due to patient recruitment issue. However, the trend suggests a beneficial effect in adding oral aciclovir to the treatment of HSV iridocyclitis in patients receiving topical corticosteroid.

16. J. There is no benefit prescribing oral aciclovir treatment for herpes zoster ophthalmicus patient post-vesicle eruption phase. Despite some textbooks describe oral treatment is not beneficial beyond 72 hours of the onset of the skin lesions, the pre-vesicle phase may last

longer than this, the patient may benefit from treatment. Unlike in herpes simplex keratitis, oc. acyclovir is not indicated in herpes zoster keratitis.

17. E. Soft shell technique (dispersive viscoelastic to coat the corneal endothelium and cohesive viscoelastic to maintain the anterior chamber) and judicious use of ultrasound energy during phacoemulsification are helpful to reduce the incidence of postoperative corneal oedema.

18. G. Despite the risk factors for this feared complication includes diabetes, high myopia and raised IOP, the most severe factor from the option list is the high systolic BP. The condition occurs due to haemorrhage into the suprachoiroidal space after rupture of a short or long ciliary artery. In severe cases, the IOP is so high that the intraocular contents are pushed out of the surgical incision, hence the name expulsive haemorrhage.

19. E. The intermittent blurring is secondary to a spike in the IOP. The chafing of the posterior segment of the iris against the lens causes the iris transillumination defect. During strenuous exercise, there is a sudden release of pigments causing a pigment storm. The incidence of PDS decreases with age due to age-related miosis and lens enlargement, which results in relative pupillary block lifting the peripheral iris away from the lens zonules.

20. B. Epithelial downgrowth is a rare condition nowadays. In the early 20th century, up to 20% of enucleations after cataract extraction were secondary to this condition. It typically presents a few months after the initial surgery or trauma. The corneal epithelium must gain entry into the eye, as it does not develop de novo within the eye by metaplasia. Epithelial downgrowth is commonly caused by persistent leaky wound, which may allow conjunctival or corneal epithelium to grow over normal intraocular tissue, including the corneal endothelium, iris and angle structures. The mechanism of glaucoma is usually a combination of PAS causing synechial closure, persistent uveitis and trabeculum obstruction by the invading epithelium.

21. E. Management of choroidal melanoma depends on the patient (age, systemic metastasis, health, wishes) and tumour (size, location, tumour extension, state of fellow eye) factors. Brachytherapy is the most appropriate treatment to preserve as much useful vision as possible in this patient. Tumour of up to 5mm thick can be treated with ruthenium plaque and up to 10mm with iodine plaque.

22. H. The presence of rubeosis and a shallow anterior chamber suggest extensive involvement of the ciliary body. The tumour is too thick for radiotherapy and the base too wide for surgical resection.

23. J. The patient can be observed. Up to a quarter of patients have spontaneous resolution of detached retina. Laser photocoagulation can be considered if the visual acuity is affected. Pars plana vitrectomy and gas tamponade are performed should laser fails.

24. F. The patient has uveal effusion syndrome. The primary abnormality is in the sclera, with secondary effects on transcleral protein permeability and compression of the vortex veins. The most common surgical treatment is a 5-7 mm sclerostomy down to the choroid to allow egress of the proteinaceous fluid. This is repeated in all four quadrants producing direct fistulae between the suprachoroidal and subtenon spaces. The dissected conjunctivae are pulled over the sclerostomies and secured. Vortex vein decompression has also been shown to be effective.

25. E. The ocular signs of sympathetic ophthalmia and VKH are not dissimilar. However the latter usually has extraocular signs e.g. hearing loss, headache and vitiligo. It's highly unlike for sympathetic ophthalmia to occur without any past ophthalmic history.

26. G. Sarcoidosis is the likely diagnosis. Tuberculosis and sarcoidosis have very similar presentations. Both conditions can cause periphlebitis and choroiditis, however only sarcoidosis causes preretinal granulomata (Lander's sign). Birdshot chorioretinopathy and multifocal choiroiditis with panuveitis do not affect the retinal veins.

27. C. The Hummelsheim procedure involves disinserting the lateral halves of the superior and inferior recti and reattaching them above and below the lateral rectus. The medial rectus is recessed. Another surgical option is the Jensen procedure where the superior, inferior and lateral recti are split into halves about 15mm from their insertions without disinsertion. The halves are tied loosely together in pairs. The main advantage of this method is to reduce the risk of anterior segment ischaemic from disinsertion of the recti.

28. A. This patient has left monocular elevator deficit. The cause is thought to be either supranuclear in origin, a tight inferior rectus or hypoplastic superior rectus. Base-up prism is appropriate if there is no abnormal head posture. However in the case, surgery is indicated. Knapp procedure involves detachment and reinsertion of medial and lateral recti along the medial and lateral borders of the superior rectus. Inverse Knapp is for correction of inferior rectus palsy.

29. F. This is dyskeratosis which is keratinisation within the dermis rather than hyperkeratosis which is increases thickness on the epidermis. The likely diagnosis is an epidermoid cyst. Keratoacanthoma exhibits hyperkeratosis as well as dyskeratosis surrounded by thickened squamous epithelium.

30. G. Schwann cells are only found in nervous tissue. Solitary neurofibroma can occur in adults and only 25% are associated with neurofibromatosis type 1.

31. B. Nasopharyngeal carcinoma is more common in oriental patients. The sixth nerve paresis and nasal symptoms are suggestive of this condition. Acoustic neuromas usually present with hearing loss and corneal anaesthesia.

32. G. The presence of Horner syndrome and involvement of the third and sixth nerves point to a cavernous sinus disorder. The lack of conjunctival hyperaemia rules out carotid-cavernous fistula. The most likely diagnosis is intracavernous carotid aneurysm. If this ruptures, it forms a high-flow carotid-cavernous fistula.

33. C. Classical angina is provoked by exertion, especially after a meal or in the cold and is usually aggravated by emotional excitement. Unstable angina refers to angina of recent onset, worsening angina or angina at rest. During an attack, ST depression and T wave inversion may appear. Variant angina occurs without provocation as a result of coronary spasm, and with characteristic ST elevation.

34. F. The patient has an anaphylactic shock due to fluorescein. The incidence is about 1 in 19000.

35. C. Central or paracentral stromal thinning is the hallmark of keratoconus.

36. E. The deposits are amyloid with can also be confirmed with Congo red.

37. D. The BOLT study showed that intravitreal bevacizumab has better outcome than macular laser in treating diabetic macular oedema. Triamcinolone has worse results compared to modified ETDRS macular laser treatment as found in the DRCR.net. Macular ischaemia is unlikely with this level of visual acuity.

38. H. This patient requires urgent vitrectomy to clear the premacular subhyaloid haemorrhage. Prolonged exposure to the blood is likely to cause irreversible toxic effect of the retina. If vitrectomy cannot be arranged YAG vitreolysis may be attempted in experienced hands however may prove difficult with coexisting vitreous haemorrhage.

39. I. There signs are due to a supraorbital mass. The dystopia, proptosis and reduced sensation of the forehead provide vital clue to this. The superior and inferior branches of the third nerve exiting the orbital apex are displaced downward and stretched, causing *forme fruste* third nerve palsy.

40. G. This is a high-flow carotid-cavernous fistula. The symptoms are secondary to III, IV, V_{1-2}, and VI nerves palsy. The bilaterality of engorged conjunctival vessels is due to increased venous return.

41. H. A topical beta-blocker is indicated. The prostaglandin analogues are not suitable due to the anterior uveitis. Brimonidine can precipitate a hypertensive crisis with tricyclic antidepressants. Brinzolamide may exacerbate the corneal oedema.

42. D. Brimonidine is an α_2-agonist. It stimulates the Muller muscle therefore improving the ptosis.

43. B. The size of the defect warrants a Hughes flap. However, the patient only has one good eye and the second stage of the operation can only take place about 6 - 10 weeks later. In this case, a posterior lamellar graft with skin mobilisation is preferred. A graft should preferably be covered by local vascularised flap to ensure good blood supply. The graft can be obtained from the fellow upper lid. Tenzel flap is only suitable if the horizontal defect is less than 70%.

44. E. Periosteal flap provides a good anchor for repair of the upper tarsus and lateral canthal tendon excision. A free posterior lamellar graft will not provide adequate support.

45. A. Despite this condition is rare, it is the most common immunobullous disease seen in children. There is a tendency for new blisters to occur in a ring around old ones ('string of beads') and small blisters to group together ('cluster of jewels'). The blisters are subepidermis rather than within the epidermis (e.g. pemphigus). When presenting in adult, the limbs are most likely to be affected first. Linear IgA is idiopathic and skin biopsy is diagnostic. Bullous pemphigoid does not usually affect the mucosa unless mucous membrane pemphigoid occurs in association.

46. C. In Stevens-Johnson syndrome, the disease is restricted to mucosa surfaces and milder bullous involvement of the skin. On the other hand, toxic epidermal necrolysis is characterised by widespread blistering with sloughing of more than 30% of the skin. Fever, epithelial surface involvement of the lungs, bladder, and gastrointestinal tract are common. Toxic epidermal necrolysis is more

serious than Stevens-Johnson syndrome. Multiorgan failure and sepsis often occurs with a mortality rate of up to 50%.

47. A. The ACCORD trial showed that fenofibrate is effective in preventing progression of established diabetic retinopathy in type 2 diabetes. It should be considered for patients with pre-proliferative diabetic retinopathy and/or diabetic maculopathy, particularly in those with macular oedema requiring laser. The FIELD study investigated the impact of fenofibrate on the progression of diabetic eye disease. Although this was not significant for the entire cohort, it was significant among patients with pre-existing retinopathy. The ADVANCE trial showed that better blood pressure control (with a combination blood-pressure lowering treatment) failed to significantly impact on the rate of retinopathy deterioration or need for laser treatment compared with conventional control. CARDS showed that atorvastatin 10mg daily resulted in a trend to reduction of laser therapy compared with placebo, but no influence on diabetic retinopathy progression.

48. E. The DIRECT study failed to show any statistical significant difference in the progression of established retinopathy in type 1 diabetes by candesartan. However, in type 2 patients there was significantly greater regression of established diabetic retinopathy in the treatment group. Regression was noted in patients with mild, but not in those with moderate or more severe diabetic retinopathy. Candesartan had no effect on the incidence of proliferative retinopathy or macular oedema. This supports the concept that once capillary closure and ischaemia is extensive, medical therapies may have less impact on the progression of diabetic retinopathy. In the EUCLID trial, lisinopril showed a non-significant reduction in incidence of retinopathy, however a significant reduction in the progression of diabetic retinopathy over 2 years. RASS showed similar results with enalapril or losartan over 5 years. The HOPE trial showed a non-significant relative risk reduction in diabetic patients requiring retinal laser treatment.

49. D. Pernicious anaemia is an autoimmune disorder in which there is loss of parietal cells in the gastric mucosa causing malabsorption of vitamin B_{12}.

50. A. This is a major cause of blindness in young children in the world. Xerophthalmia has been classified by WHO. Impaired visual adaptation followed by nyctalopia is the first symptom. There is dryness and thickening of the conjunctiva and cornea. Bitot's spots (white plaques of keratinized epithelial cells) are found on the

conjunctiva. These spots can, however be seen without vitamin A deficiency, secondary by harsh environment exposure. Keratomalacia eventually occurs with increased risk of infective keratitis and blindness.

51. H. This is cytomegalovirus retinitis. The initial management should be intravenous ganciclovir before changing to oral treatment when the disease improves. Intravitreal ganciclovir is usually used to assess the temporary response prior to slow-release ganciclovir implant, and is not suitable for possible systemic cytomegalovirus infection such as in this case.

52. D. The patient has intermediate uveitis. Topical steroid is unlikely to be beneficial. Patients can be started on oral prednisolone however posterior subtenon triamcinolone has the advantage of reducing systemic side-effect of steroid.

53. B. Early hypofluorescence and late hyperfluorescence is the hallmark of white dot syndrome. However, only birdshot retinochoroidopathy causes optic disc hyperfluorescence. Macula hyperfluorescence may also occur due to cystoids macula oedema.

54. F. The lipofuscin deposits in the RPE layer block the fluorescence from the dye. The late hyperfluorescence is due to macula atrophic defect in Stargardt disease.

55. H. This patient has Schwartz-Mazuo syndrome. The RPE cells released from retinal tears and detachment block the trabecular meshwork causing the IOP rise. The condition usually resolves after the retinal detachment is repaired.

56. I. The corneal defect is due to posterior polymorphous dystrophy. This condition is associated with Alport syndrome, which is a hereditary nephritis with haematuria. Progression to renal failure is common. Patients also have sensorineural deafness. Posterior polymorphous dystrophy may be confused with iridocorneal endothelial syndrome. The latter is almost always unilateral.

57. A. Thayer-Martin medium is specific to gram negative cocci. MacConkey contains lactose, therefore only lactose fermenting gram negative can grow on it. Blood agar is suitable for most bacteria but does not detect haemophilus, neisseria or moraxella. It is important to combine it with chocolate agar, which theses bacteria will grow on. Cooked meat broth is used for anaerobe and fastidious organism. Aerobes grow on the surface and anaerobes inside the thioglycate agar.

58. J. The McCoy medium is used to detect this obligate intracellular bacterium. The non-nutrient agar with *E.coli* is for acanthamoeba, and Sabouraud for fungi. Lowerstein-Jensen medium is used for *mycoplasma tuberculosis.*

59. D. The symptoms are due lateral medullary and cerebellar syndrome. An acute episode usually presents with sudden unsteadiness (cerebellar ataxia), facial pain (trigeminal nerve) and hoarseness (glossopharyngeal nerve). Ocular signs are Horner syndrome, cerebellar syndrome related (e.g. nystagmus, ocular dysmetria). There can also be sensory loss and hemiparesis on the contralateral side.

60. F. The signs are suggestive of a dorsal midbrain syndrome. The neurons that participate in vergence eye movements are located in this region, therefore patients with vertical palsy often have deficits on convergence, with exotropia for near, and esotropia for distant. Convergence-retraction nystagmus can be demonstrated using an optokinetic drum. Skew deviation results from supranuclear dysfunction and has no localising value. The ability to elevate the eyes reduces with advanced age. Patients over the age of 80 may only be capable of half the range of younger subjects.

61. I. Membranous cataract is rare and usually seen in Hallerman-Streiff syndrome. Majority of patients have dental abnormality and proportionate dwarfism. Other diagnostic features include hypotrichosis and atrophy of skin especially on the nose. The gene defect lacks a hereditary pattern and most reported cases suggest sporadic mutations. Aicardi is also not an inherited condition. There is usually high mortality rate if inherited by males. The condition causes corpus collosum agenesis (causing infantile spasm), choroidal lacunae, optic disc hypoplasia, microphthalmos and persistent pupillary membrane. Allagille syndrome is inherited as an autosomal dominant condition. The deletion defect in the inherited gene causes disrupt signalling pathway during embryonic development. The patients usually presents with optic disc drusen, posterior embryotoxon, jaundice (reduced bile duct) and tetralogy of Fallot. CHARGE represents **C**oloboma, **H**eart defect, choanal **A**tresia, **R**etarted growth, **G**enital and **E**ar defects. Cornelia de Lange syndrome consists of microcornea, synophyr, low hairline, developmental and muscloskeletal abnormalities. De Morsier syndrome patients usually have optic disc hypoplasia, agenesis of septum pellucidum with malformation of corpus collosum and hypothalamic dysfunction (causing stunted growth).

62. J. Lowe syndrome is an X-linked inborn error of <u>amino acid</u> metabolism. Ninety-five percent of amino acids are usually reabsorbed in the renal tubules, however in this condition aminoaciduria occurs due to reabsorption defect. Galactosaemia is another form of inborn error of amino acid metabolism which commonly presents with cataract. Fabry disease is an X-linked disease caused by a deficiency in α-galactosidase A. Excess accumulation of lysosomal material ensues, causing peripheral neuropathy, gastrointestinal symptoms and eventually cardiac and renal diseases. Patients typically have vortex-keratopathy, wedge-shaped cataract and ocular vessel tortuosity.

63. B. The shallow anterior chamber and low IOP suggest either an underproduction of aqueous or over-drainage. There absence of leakage and a flat bleb point to the former. Ciliary body shutdown is not uncommon post-trabeculectomy and usually recovers soon after. In this case, the condition does not require further intervention unless there is hypotonous maculopathy. The patient should be followed-up closely.

64. F. The signs support the diagnosis of aqueous misdirection. Topical cycloplegic is indicated before anterior vitreous YAG laser or surgical intervention. Suprachoroidal haemorrhage presents with similar anterior segment signs and may be missed without adequate fundoscopy. The latter may require urgent drainage to preserve sight.

65. A. The signs strongly suggest ocular ischaemic syndrome. Auscultation of the carotid arteries and heart should be performed. An urgent carotid Doppler ultrasound is required to assess the patency of the artery and an echocardiogram should also be requested.

66. E. A CT head is warranted to assess the amount of orbital damage. MRI is contraindicated due to the possibility of a metal foreign body in the orbit. A skull X-ray does not provide adequate information about the ocular tissue status.

67. E. The Lincoff rule suggests in a bullous inferior retinal detachment, the break usually lies above the horizontal meridian. However, if the retinal break is close to the 12 o'clock position, the superior retinal is also likely to be detached.

68. A. When the entire superior retinal is detached, the defect is usually near the 12 o'clock position. Retinoschitic related detachment does not undulate. It involves tears in the inner and outer layer. Macular hole can cause macular detachment. The aetiology can be traumatic or following the resolution of commotion retinae.

69. E. The recommended guideline is simultaneous treatment. Separate sets of instruments should be used for each eye. The patient should be made aware of the usual cumulative risks of sequential injections either to each eye on separate visits or to both eyes on the same visit.

70. H. The College recommends that an elevated IOP even of more than 30mmHg, should not preclude treatment provided the IOP is treated simultaneously.

71. C. The likely diagnosis is early onset esotropia. The angle of deviation is large and similar for near and distant. The refractive error is usually normal for the age of the child. Inferior oblique overaction is common, and can present concurrently or later.

72. G. Paretic esotropia has incomitant deviation and a greater deviation for distant than for near. Children and young adults can present with isolated sixth nerve palsy post-viral infection or head trauma. A head scan is required to rule out neoplasm e.g. brain glioma.

73. D. Optic nerve glioma frequently presents in childhood. It can cause central retinal vein occlusion. CT scan is a helpful investigation to differentiate between optic glioma and meningioma. Many optic gliomas are associated with good visual function for the lifetime of the patient. Thus, the lesion is not treated unless there is indication of progressive visual loss or proptosis. Chemotherapy is usually recommended for young children. Older children and adult undergo conventional radiotherapy. Surgical removal of the optic glioma is not possible without removing the optic nerve. Therefore this option is only indicated for severe proptosis or extension of the tumour towards the optic chiasm.

74. F. Neuroblastoma is a tumour of early childhood. About 20% of patients have orbital metastasis. Neuroblastoma originates in the adrenal medulla or the paraspinal sites where sympathetic nervous system tissue is present. Proptosis and periorbital ecchymosis ('raccoon eyes') are common and arise from retrobulbar metastases. Extensive bone marrow metastases may result in pancytopenia and therefore subconjunctival haemorrhages.

75. B. Erythromycin and clarithromycin are not recommended to be prescribed to patients on simvastatin. There is also increased risk of myopathy with patient on atorvastatin and erythromycin. Other types of statin are not known to have the same risk.

76. G. Tamsulosin is an α_1-antagonist. Patients on this treatment can have intraoperative floppy iris syndrome. Alfuzosin, doxazosin, terazosin and prazosin may also cause this phenomenon.

77. B. This patient is very likely to have an intraorbital haemorrhage. Waiting for a CT scan to be performed is likely to compromise his vision further. An urgent lateral canthotomy should be considered.

78. J. Medial wall fracture does not require repair unless the medial rectus is entrapped. The cause for this patient's diplopia is likely due to the tissue oedema. The diplopia should improve when the swelling subsides. However, the patient should be followed-up until his symptoms have resolved.

79. A. The diagnostic criteria for Kearn-Sayre syndrome are progressive external ophthalmoplegia, pigmentary retinopathy and onset at less than 20 years of age. In addition, patients must fulfilled one of the following triads – cerebellar dysfunction, cardiac conduction defects or CSF protein of >100mg/dL.

80. E. Ocular symptoms are the initial complaint in 75% of myasthenia gravis patients. Approximately 85% of patients with ocular symptoms only develop systemic disease within 2 years of diagnosis. The onset of diplopia may be insidious or abrupt, frequently intermittent with irregular intervals of occurrence. Ptosis is often asymmetrical.

81. C. Groenblad-Strandberg syndrome is a combination of pseudoxanthoma elasticum and angioid streaks. Despite the skin defect, patients with pseudoxanthoma elasticum usually presents with non-dermatological problems e.g. gastrointestinal bleed, early myocardial infarction, claudication or renal dysfunction.

82. H. Tuberous sclerosis (a.k.a Bourneville disease or Pringle disease) is an autosomal dominant phacomatosis. Patients have hamartomas in multiple organs which may not present until late childhood. This condition has numerous types of cutaneous lesions in the form of adenoma sebaceum, ash leaf hypopigmentation, shagreen patches (cutaneous plaques), skin tags and cafe-au-lait spots. Internal hamartomas can occur in the heart, lungs, kidneys, brain and retinae. Asymptomatic family members of a suspected patient should be carefully examined under UV light as they may have harbour 'forme fruste' of the condition which can manifest just as hypopigmented patches. This and gonadal mosaicism may have genetic implications for future offspring.

83. E. A multicenter study is the most suitable method when the condition is rare and no single medical centre has access to a sufficient number of patients to reach a valid conclusion in a reasonable time period. It can solve the problem of inadequate sample size, and if multiple centres with somewhat different patients

and physicians reach a conclusion on a given treatment, it tends to increase confidence in the results. A common protocol needs to be developed where all the participating centres agree on patient management. Since medical centres have a propensity to have their own management method and data collection, multicenter studies require considerable negotiation to get agreement on a single set of procedures.

84. B. There are a few way to grade the strength of medical evidence. The alphabetical grading scale is similar to the Roman numeral grading scale, except the latter has sub-grades and is more elaborate.

85. H. Toxocariasis can present with an inflamed or quiet eye. In younger children, *toxoplasma canis* can cause chronic endophthalmitis. In older children, a quiet posterior or peripheral granuloma with or without associated traction vitreoretinal band may be present. Treatment involves anti-helminthic and systemic steroid (if ocular inflammation is present).

86. B. Coat disease presents in childhood. It is non-hereditary and about 90% of the cases are unilateral. Intraretinal exudates can track away from the area of retinal telangiectasia. Argon laser to the abnormal vessel region is indicated for progressive exudation, and vitreoretinal intervention for retinal detachment.

87. D. A similar question was asked in the EMQ paper in February 2011. Some of the migraine auras are known as scintillating scotoma (blind spot with shimmering border), fortification spectrum (angular lines aura) and palinopsia (persistence of a part or entire image after the object is removed from the patient's visual field). Moore's lighting streak is the temporal streak of light seen in dim environment by patients with vitreous detachment. Haidinger brush refers to a visual phenomenon where a yellowish bow-tie shape with fuzzy ends (hence the term 'brush') is seen in polarized blue light. Phosphene is the bright light defect perceived by patients with optic nerve or retina dysfunction. It can also be induced by firm rubbing of closed eyes.

88. G. This is Riddoch phenomenon which is caused by lesions in the occipital lobe. It limits the sufferer's ability to distinguish objects. Moving objects are not perceived to have color or shape. There may be awareness of the movement without perception of it (agnosanopsia). The patient may deny blindness (Anton syndrome). The Pulfrich phenomenon refers to the discrepancy between images perceived by the optic nerves, with one slightly damaged. It causes the image to move in a strange way e.g. when a unilateral optic

neuritis patient observes a pendulum moving in one plane with both eyes, the motion seems like elliptical.

89. B. Bardet-Biedl syndrome is inherited in an autosomal recessive fashion. The retinitis pigmentosa is severe and most patients are severely sight impaired in their twenties. Alstrom syndrome patients have hyperinsulinaemia, hyperlipidaemia and sensorineural deafness. Cockayne syndrome, like most conditions related to retinitis pigmentosa, is inherited autosomal recessively. Patients have photophobia, hearing loss, bird-like facies and progeric dwarfism.

90. I. Refsum syndrome is an inborn error of metabolism with deficiency in phytanic acid hydroxylase enzyme. The excess phytanic acid permeates various body tissues. Unlike most conditions associated with retinitis pigmentosa, this is treatable with plasmapheresis to remove the circulating phytanic acid and a phytanic acid-free diet. Bassen-Kornzweig syndrome is caused by deficiency in β-lipoprotein resulting in intestinal malabsorption. Patients have cerebellar ataxia and progressive ophthalmoplegia. Blood film showing acanthocytosis is diagnostic. Treatment is with vitamin E.

MCQ Paper 2

1) Which is not a contraindication to indocyanine green angiography?
   a. pregnancy
   b. uraemia
   c. seafood allergy
   d. breast feeding

2) The following drugs cause accommodative disturbance except
   a. amitriptyline
   b. amiodarone
   c. neostigmine
   d. levodopa

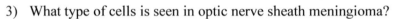

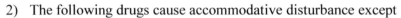

3) What type of cells is seen in optic nerve sheath meningioma?
   a. Schaumann bodies
   b. psammoma bodies
   c. verocay bodies
   d. asteroid bodies

4) Which is incorrect regarding Nd:YAG laser?
   a. it emits infrared radiation
   b. the laser wavelength is invisible to the naked eye
   c. the pulsed laser creates plasma
   d. the laser device is fitted with lithium/neon beam

5) Stevens-Johnson syndrome is the result of which type of hypersensitivity reaction?
   a. I
   b. II
   c. III
   d. IV

6) Which condition can cause a central Horner syndrome?
   a. syringomyelia
   b. carotid aneurysm
   c. carotid-cavernous fistula
   d. nasopharyngeal carcinoma

7) Which feature is associated with iridocorneal endothelial syndrome?
   a. posterior embryotoxon
   b. iris stromal atrophy
   c. iris strands to Schwalbe line
   d. rubeosis iridis

8) The optical defects below are secondary to the prismatic effect at the edge of a convex lens except
   a. spherical aberration
   b. ring scotoma
   c. pin cushion effect
   d. barrel effect

9) Which vector causes onchocerciasis?
   a. Chrysops (horse fly)
   b. Simulium (black fly)
   c. Sand fly
   d. Ixodes tick

10) The following structures pass through the superior orbital fissure except
   a. trochlear nerve
   b. abducen nerve
   c. ophthalmic artery
   d. superior ophthalmic vein

11) Which is a feature of fully accommodative esotropia?
   a. the esotropia is fully corrected by glasses
   b. the AC/A ratio is high
   c. amblyopia is usually present
   d. the magnitude of deviation between near and distance usually >15PD

12) A HIV patient presents with choroiditis and periphlebitis. The fluorescent treponemal antibodies absorbed test is positive. What is the appropriate antibiotic treatment for this patient?
    a. metronidazole
    b. sulfadiazine
    c. penicillin
    d. gentamicin

13) Which statement is true regarding cancer-associated retinopathy?
    a. visual symptoms almost always present after the diagnosis of malignancy
    b. there is usually visual acuity deterioration without colour desaturation
    c. the condition is usually bilateral
    d. the initial symptoms are secondary to rod dysfunction

14) The following genes are implicated in retinitis pigmentosa except
    a. rhodopsin
    b. peripherin
    c. ROM1
    d. ABCA4

15) Which is true regarding the numbers below?
        4, 4, 6, 8, 9, 11
    a. the median is 8
    b. the mode is 5
    c. the mean is 6
    d. the standard deviation is $\sqrt{8}$

16) Which condition is not associated with peripheral ulcerative keratitis?
    a. rheumatoid arthritis
    b. Wegener granulomatosis
    c. primary Sjogren syndrome
    d. relapsing polychondritis

17) A 25-year-old high myope presents with a macular-on inferior retinal detachment without a Weiss ring. A retinal tear is noted inferiorly. What is the most appropriate surgical management?
    a. vitrectomy
    b. scleral buckling
    c. combined vitrectomy and scleral buckling
    d. vitrectomy and silicone oil

18) According to the Royal College of Ophthalmologists guideline for cataract surgery, which of the following is incorrect?
    a. patient at risk of developing cystoids macular oedema should be considered for topical non-steroidal anti-inflammatory treatment pre- and post-cataract operation
    b. if the departmental endophthalmitis rate is higher than that of published in the Bolton study (0.055%), then intracameral cefuroxime should be considered
    c. the main corneal section should be sutured in children
    d. intravenous access is not required for peribulbar anaesthetic

19) Which is correct regarding MRI T1 tissue signal intensity?
    a. fat > white matter > gray matter > CSF
    b. CSF > gray matter > white matter > fat
    c. fat > gray matter > white matter > CSF
    d. CSF = gray matter > white matter > fat

20) The enzyme activity of thiopurine methyltransferase (TPMT) is usually checked before the commencement of which drug?
    a. methotrexate
    b. azathioprine
    c. cyclophosphamide
    d. ciclosporin

21) The following methods are employed to reduce confounding factors except
    a. randomisation
    b. patient matching
    c. stratified analysis
    d. increasing the sample size

22) Which statement is incorrect regarding intraocular pressure?
   a. it decreases with age
   b. it always displays a diurnal rhythm
   c. extreme position of gazes causing an increase in the IOP
   d. decreases when sleeping

23) The following infections can cause congenital cataract except
   a. rubella
   b. herpes simplex
   c. tuberculosis
   d. HIV

24) Which structure does not derived from the mesoderm?
   a. endothelium of blood vessels
   b. superotemporal connective tissue
   c. striated extraocular muscles
   d. corneal stroma

25) Which description does not apply to congenital nystagmus?
   a. it is accentuated by fixating at near object
   b. the nystagmus is minimal at the null position
   c. manifests reversed optokinetic nystagmus
   d. it is associated with nystagmus blocking syndrome

26) Based on the General Medical Council (UK) guidance on consent, which of the following apply to a 14-year-old with a ruptured globe trauma proposed for a primary repair?
   a. he can presumed to have the capacity to consent
   b. both parents are required to consent for the procedure
   c. the operation can proceed in the patient's best interest without parental consent
   d. the parents can override his refusal to consent even if he has the capacity to consent

27) The following statements are true about blepharochalasis apart from
    a. it usually presents in teenagers
    b. it is an inflammatory disorder
    c. the lower eyelids may be affected
    d. it is usually painless

28) Which index on the Humphrey visual field test provides an indication of the degree of generalised loss in the visual field compared to age-adjusted normal population values?
    a. mean deviation
    b. pattern standard deviation
    c. corrected pattern standard deviation
    d. short-term fluctuation

29) Number of cases of disease in those exposed   is defined as
            Number of individuals exposed
    a. relative risk
    b. absolute risk
    c. attributable risk
    d. odd ratio

30) Which description about irregular astigmatism is true?
    a. it usually can be corrected with glasses
    b. this is usually found in keratoconus
    c. it usually arise from the lens
    d. it cannot be corrected with refractive surgery

31) The followings are true regarding corneal topography except
    a. warm colours represent high dioptres
    b. the relative numerical scales are usually fixed
    c. it can be used to quantify corneal warping
    d. a bowtie configuration is an usual finding in most patients

32) Which sign is not seen in hypertensive retinopathy?
    a. arteriovenous nipping
    b. cotton-wool spots
    c. venous beading
    d. Elschnig spots

33) A patient is admitted for intravenous penicillin treatment for syphilis retinitis. What common reaction does the managing physician needs to be aware of?
   a. Jarisch-Herxheimer reaction
   b. anaphylactic shock
   c. disseminated intravascular coagulation
   d. severe anaemia

34) Which sign does not occur in left aberrant regeneration of the third nerve?
   a. left pupil constriction on downgaze
   b. retraction of the left eyelid on attempted adduction
   c. left pupil usually reacts normally to light
   d. left suppressed vertical optokinetic response

35) Select the correct description for the electroretinogram.
   a. the b-wave is produced by the retinal pigment epithelial cells
   b. the b-wave is maximal with a bright white flash stimulus in photopic conditions
   c. can be used to distinguish between macular and optic nerve diseases
   d. cone dystrophy has abnormal 30Hz flickers

36) Which is incorrect regarding the image formed by a prism?
   a. erect
   b. virtual
   c. displaced towards the apex
   d. diminished

37) The following descriptions are correct about an acute inflammatory respond except
   a. it is non-specific
   b. it is non-adaptive
   c. the vascular permeability decreases
   d. it is initiated by a vascular phase followed by cellular phase

38) The synoptophore can be used to investigate the following except
   a. the degree of stereopsis
   b. vertical and torsional misalignments simultaneously
   c. sensory fusion
   d. abnormal retinal correspondence

39) Which of the following statement is true regarding steroid-induced raised IOP?
   a. it is always reversible with cessation of the steroid
   b. there is increased risk with pigmentary glaucoma
   c. is more common in patients with hypermetropia
   d. may present within 3 days of starting hourly topical steroid

40) Which nerve do the sympathetic fibres travel in the orbit?
   a. nasociliary nerve
   b. frontal nerve
   c. optic nerve
   d. superior branch of the third nerve

41) Which investigations are unlikely to yield useful information for a patient suspected to have sarcoidosis?
   a. serum angiotensin-converting enzyme
   b. serum calcium
   c. creatinine kinase
   d. C-reactive protein

42) The following statements regarding herpes simplex virus 1 are true except
   a. it is a double stranded DNA virus
   b. cornea stromal disease is caused by replicating virus
   c. latent virus resides in the trigeminal ganglion
   d. can be auto-inoculated at site of trauma and presents as blisters

43) Which of the following does not apply to all lasers?
   a. monochromatic
   b. coherent
   c. collimated
   d. polarised

44) Which statement is incorrect regarding an X-linked recessive disease?
   a. the disease is transmitted from the affected male to all his sons
   b. if a female carrier has children with a normal male, half of her daughters will be carriers
   c. all daughters of an affected males are carriers
   d. the disease is only manifested in a female if the gene is in homozygous state

45) How many clearly identifiable peaks should a good ultrasound contact A-scan have in a phakic eye?
   a. four
   b. five
   c. six
   d. seven

46) The following descriptions are true for pilocarpine except
   a. it can be used to treat accommodative esotropia
   b. causes brow ache
   c. constricts an atropine mydriasis
   d. constricts a phenylephrine mydriasis

47) Which condition is usually not associated with retinal detachment?
   a. Pseudoxanthoma elasticum
   b. Stickler syndrome
   c. Marfan syndrome
   d. Ehlers-Danlos syndrome

48) The possible histological findings of rhabdomyosarcoma are listed below except
   a. embryonal
   b. alveolar
   c. pleomorphic
   d. spindle

49) For a patient involved in a road traffic accident, the following details should be recorded for medicolegal consideration except
   a. the name of the person driving the vehicle
   b. eyewitness statement
   c. the name of the person who administered first aid treatment
   d. the names of the police officers involved

50) Which is not found in the human tear?
   a. IgA
   b. IgD
   c. IgM
   d. IgG

51) The recommendations of the Royal College of Ophthalmologists guideline in preventing post-cataract operation endophthalmitis include
   a. povidine iodine 5% solution to be instilled in the conjunctival sac prior to surgery
   b. subconjunctival injection of antibiotic at the end of the surgery
   c. treat blepharitis, conjunctivitis and nasolacrimal infections prior to surgery.
   d. reject lens implants which have inadvertently contacted the lid margins

52) Which statement is incorrect regarding tuberculosis?
   a. primary tuberculosis is symptomless in majority of patients
   b. it is a notifiable disease in the UK
   c. the Mantoux test is almost always positive in severe tuberculosis
   d. the chest X-ray usually shows patchy nodular shadows in the upper zones of the lungs in pulmonary tuberculosis

53) Which issue is not addressed in the economic evaluation of a health care program?
   a. allocative efficiency
   b. technical efficiency
   c. effectiveness efficiency
   d. requirement efficiency

54) What type of cataract is associated with atopic dermatitis?
    a. anterior subcapsular shield cataract
    b. anterior capsular sun-flower cataract
    c. stellate posterior subcapsular cataract
    d. posterior cortical cataract

55) A patient presents with acute right homonymous hemianopia. What is the best imaging study for the patient?
    a. MRI
    b. CT
    c. MR angiogram
    d. CT angiogram

56) Where is the most likely site of dysfunction in blepharospasm?
    a. facial nerve root near the cerebellopontine angle
    b. facial nucleus in pons
    c. basal ganglia
    d. orbicularis oculi

57) Which statement is incorrect regarding argon laser trabeculoplasty?
    a. the laser burns are placed at the junction of the pigmented and non-pigmented section of the trabecular meshwork
    b. is more effective in Black patients
    c. is more effective in patients with pseudoexfoliation glaucoma
    d. the failure rate is 30% at 5 years

58) Select the true description about tyrosinase-negative albinism.
    a. it is an autosomal dominant condition
    b. there are more crossed optic nerve fibres at the optic chiasm
    c. stereopsis is usually present
    d. patients do not usually have squint

59) Cataract can be induced by the drugs below except
    a. allopurinol
    b. phenothiazide
    c. chloroquine
    d. amiodarone

60) The following conditions can be caused by herpes zoster except
    a. trichiasis
    b. neurotrophic keratitis
    c. disciform keratitis
    d. peripheral ulcerative keratitis

61) Which statement is correct regarding the Hess chart obtained from a Lees screen test?
    a. the bigger chart indicates the eye with the paretic muscle
    b. the smaller chart indicates the overacting eye
    c. with the passage of time, the charts in both eyes become more concomitant
    d. each square on the chart represents about 5 prism diopter

62) What is responsible for acute extraocular muscle oedema in thyroid orbitopathy?
    a. glycosaminoglycans
    b. keratin deposition
    c. hypertrophy of blood vessels
    d. hypertrophy of myocytes

63) Which statement is true regarding congenital fibrosis of extraocular muscles?
    a. the condition is usually progressive
    b. the eyes are usually anchored in downgaze
    c. there is rarely any issue with abduction
    d. the average age of onset is 5 years

64) According to the Royal College of Ophthalmologists screening guidelines for patients on vigabatrin, which of the following strategies is advocated?
    a. a base line visual acuity and colour vision should be performed at the start of treatment
    b. visual field test should be performed every year for the first 3 years
    c. threshold perimetry testing is recommended to detect early defect
    d. visual field test up to 45 degrees of eccentricity should be performed

65) Which infection is unlikely to occur in a HIV patient with a CD4+ count of 300/μl?
   a. herpes zoster
   b. tuberculosis uveitis
   c. toxoplasmosis
   d. aspergillosis

66) In a hypothesis test of the IOP mean between two treatment groups , if α = 0.05, the correct statement is
   a. an incorrect inference is made 95% of the time
   b. there is a 5% chance of inferring a real difference when there is none
   c. there is a 5% chance of inferring no real difference when there is one
   d. 95% of the time the null hypothesis will be correct

67) Indocyanine green angiography provides more information than fundus fluorescein angiogram in the circumstances mentioned except
   a. predominant classic choroidal neovascular membrane
   b. choroidal neovascular membrane associated with an overlying haemorrhage
   c. in retinal angiomatous proliferation
   d. in idiopathic polypoidal choroidal vasculopathy

68) The following drugs can cause optic neuropathy except
   a. ethambutol
   b. isoniazid
   c. rifampicin
   d. chloramphenicol

69) Which statement is true regarding basal cell carcinoma?
   a. it is more commonly found on the upper than the lower lid
   b. the tumour arises from the basal cells of the dermis
   c. it frequently metastasises
   d. the tumours that recurs tend to be more aggressive

70) The most immature cells found in retinoblastoma is
   a. Homer-Wright rosettes
   b. neuroblasts
   c. Flexner-Wintersteiner rosettes
   d. early retinal cells

71) Which of the white dot syndromes does not cause vitritis?
   a. birdshot retinochoroidopathy
   b. punctuate inner choroidopathy
   c. serpiginous choroidopathy
   d. acute posterior multifocal placoid pigment epitheliopathy

72) What is the result of using unpaired t-test for paired samples?
   a. this will artificially inflate the sample size
   b. there is unlikely to be any difference in the outcome
   c. the standard deviation is smaller
   d. the null hypothesis is void

73) Which investigation is unlikely to yield helpful information in a patient with myasthenia gravis?
   a. anti-acetylcholine receptor antibodies
   b. anti-striated muscle antibodies
   c. calcium-channel antibodies
   d. anti-muscle-specific receptor tyrosine kinase antibodies

74) The signs below are typical of Miller Fisher syndrome except
   a. ophthalmoplegia
   b. ataxia
   c. areflexia
   d. distal limb weakness

75) Which of the following statements is true regarding penetrating keratoplasty in the UK?
   a. 45-50% of grafts fail at the end of 5 years
   b. endothelial rejection occurs in 20-30% of grafts in 5 years
   c. 25-30% of rejection results in graft failure

d. most acute rejections occur within the first two weeks of the operation

76) The following conditions are frequently indicated for a heavy tamponade in vitreoretinal surgery except
   a. recurrent retinal detachment with extensive proliferative vitreoretinopathy
   b. traumatic retinal dialysis
   c. giant tear in the lower quadrant of the retina
   d. a high myope with a macular hole retinal detachment

77) Which statement is not true regarding topical oxybuprocaine (benoxinate)?
   a. has some degree of antimicrobial action
   b. inhibits epithelial healing
   c. has longer analgesic effect than tetracaine
   d. cannot be used systemically

78) Which form of the sickle syndromes has the mildest form of sickle-cell retinopathy?
   a. sickle cell disease
   b. sickle-cell trait
   c. sickle-cell C disease
   d. sickle-cell thalassaemia

79) Which eyelid lesion is likely to show intraepidermal proliferation of atypical spindle-shaped melanocytes on histology?
   a. lentigo maligna
   b. acquired melanocytic naevus
   c. melanoma
   d. Kaposi sarcoma

80) The following statements about pattern visual evoked potential are correct except
   a. the P100 is the largest and most reproducible component
   b. the P100 is predominantly a macula response
   c. the latency of the P100 correlates with the visual acuity
   d. demyelinating optic neuropathy produces a delay in P100

81) Which description about the chi-square (χ^2) test for two groups is false?
   a. it is used to assess whether the frequency of a condition is significantly different between the two groups
   b. all 'expected' cell frequencies should be more than 5 to provide an accurate test
   c. a large value of χ^2 indicates lack of agreement between the groups
   d. the distribution of χ^2 is Gaussian

82) The features below are only present in malignancy except
   a. poor differentiation
   b. displacing the surrounding tissue
   c. increased nuclear to cytoplasmic ratio
   d. increased heterogeneity of cells

83) A 37-year-old with binocular distant diplopia, unilateral hearing loss, facial nerve palsy and decreased corneal sensation is most likely to have
   a. dorsal midbrain disease
   b. Ramsay Hunt syndrome
   c. a cerebellopontine angle tumour
   d. Gradenigo syndrome

84) Which is an unlikely complication of silicone oil in vitrectomy?
   a. iris atrophy
   b. subconjunctival cyst formation
   c. late glaucoma
   d. filamentary keratitis

85) The following are indications for an enucleation except
   a. a blind painful eye
   b. a blind unsightly eye
   c. severe ocular trauma and a high risk for sympathetic ophthalmia
   d. refractory panophthalmitis

86) Filamentary keratitis can be caused by the conditions mentioned except
   a. blepharospasm
   b. herpes simplex keratitis
   c. Wegener granulomatosis
   d. lattice dystrophy

87) Which situation allows an abrupt cessation of systemic corticosteroids in a usually healthy patient?
   a. received 30mg daily morning doses for a month duration
   b. received 60mg daily morning doses for 3 days
   c. received 20mg daily morning doses for 3 week after stopping long-term therapy 6 months ago
   d. received 20mg daily evening doses for 2 weeks

88) The investigation least likely to yield helpful information in a malinger is
   a. Frisby test
   b. red-green duochrome chart
   c. Humphrey perimetry
   d. Goldman perimetry

89) The following are risk factors for a retinal artery occlusion except
   a. antithrombin deficiency
   b. protein S deficiency
   c. antiphospholipid syndrome
   d. carotid artery disease

90) Good practises for clinical trials exclude
   a. all patients should be followed up even if they abandon the treatment protocol
   b. patient data can be stored indefinitely after a clinical trial as long as it is done securely
   c. preparation of interim analyses based on accrued data
   d. the trial should not be stopped prematurely even after a 5% level of significance is detected

MCQ Paper 2 Answers

1) d. Breast feeding is contraindicated in FFA but not ICG. The former is secreted in breast milk. Other contraindications to ICG include iodide allergy and liver disease.

2) b. The groups of drugs known to cause accommodative disturbance include tricyclic antidepressants, anti-cholinergics and anti-parkinsonians. Amiodarone causes optic neuropathy.

3) b. Optic meningioma has two main types of cells. The other type is meningothelial. Asteroid and Schaumann bodies are seen in sarcoidosis; and verocay bodies in neurilemmoma.

4) d. The laser beam in invisible and an aiming with helium/neon is usually fitted on the device. The Nd:YAG laser emits an infrared radiation at 1064nm.

5) c. Type III with immune-complex deposits in the mucosa and skin. The most common aetiologies are drug (sulphonamides, penicillin, phenytoin), virus (herpes simplex, AIDS) and malignancies. The precipitating cause is not always identifiable.

6) a. The other conditions which can cause central Horner syndrome are diabetic autonomic neuropathy, brainstem pathology, Wallenberg syndrome and demyelinating disease. Carotid aneurysm affects the second-order neuron. Carotid-cavernous fistula and nasopharyngeal carcinoma affect the third-order neuron.

7) b. ICE syndrome is due to the proliferation of abnormal corneal endothelium. It causes a spectrum of structural changes which includes corectopia, pseudopolycoria and corneal endothelial abnormalities.

8) d. A barrel effect is caused by a thick concave lens.

9) b. The Chrysops fly carries the loa loa microfilariae. The sand fly is a vector for leishmaniasis, black fly for onchocerciasis and the *Ixodes* tick for Lyme disease (*Borrelia burgdorferi*).

10) c. The ophthalmic artery passes through the optic canal to emerge from the optic foramen.

11) a. Patients with fully accommodative esotropia usually have good binocular vision. They are relatively hypermetropic for their age and the AC/A is normal. Binocular single vision is usually present and the prognosis is generally better than for partially accommodative esotropia.

12) c. The patient has posterior uveitis likely to be due to syphilis. Mega unit dose of IV penicillin is required for treatment.

13) c. Half of the patients with CAR presents prior to the diagnosis of malignancy. The fundus appears normal in the initial stage and electrodiagnostic tests are usually required to confirm the diagnosis. The initial symptoms of acuity reduction and colour impairment are secondary to cone dysfunction. In the later stage, the rods are affected causing nyctalopia and peripheral visual loss.

14) d. The ATP-binding cassette subfamily A no. 4 (ABCA4) gene is implicated in the autosomal recessive type of Stargardt disease. In RP, different type of gene defect can cause identical and indistinguishable phenotypic manifestations. Some of the common gene mutations are in rhodopsin, peripherin and rod outer segment protein 1 (ROM1).

15) d. The standard deviation is derived from $\sqrt{\sum(X - mean)^2} / \sqrt{(n-1)}$, where X is the individual sample and n is the sample size. The median is 7, mode 4 and mean 7.

16) c. Primary Sjogren syndrome is autoimmune disease attacking the salivary and parotid glands. Other mucosa such as oral and vagina are involved too. The corneal vessels are not affected. Peripheral ulcerative keratitis is a condition secondary to ischaemic changes. The arteries supplying the cornea are end vessels, and are susceptible to occlusion from the auto-antibodies.

17) b. Scleral buckling is preferred for young phakic patients without PVD. The disadvantage of vitrectomy is the inevitable formation of cataract and subsequent loss of accommodation related to its removal. However, some surgeons may lack buckling experience and choose to perform vitrectomy with the use of silicone oil or heavy liquid. There are also disadvantages associated with scleral buckling e.g. explant related infection, extrusion, strabismus and refractive error.

18) d. Intravenous access should be established for peribulbar and retrobulbar anaesthesia. Corneal section as small as 20G equivalent is recommended to be suture with 10-0 vicryl to prevent leak and reduce the incidence of long-term induced astigmatism.

19) a. The signal intensity for 'b' applies to T2, 'c' to FLAIR and 'd' to STIR.

20) b. TMPT metabolises azathioprine. The risk of myelosuppression is increased in those with reduced activity of the enzyme.

21) d. Confounding factors can be caused by the investigators or subjects involved in the study, the instruments used in the research etc. They

result in misleading or skewed outcome. Increasing the sample size increases the power of the study to detect the difference measured. It has no impact on confounding factors.

22) a. The IOP tends to increase with age, and the causes are multifactorial e.g. increase venous return and sclerosis of the trabecular meshwork.

23) c. Intrauterine infections due to toxoplasmosis, rubella, CMV, herpes simplex and zoster and HIV (forms the acronym TORCH) are known to cause congenital cataract.

24) d. The corneal stroma and the rest of the connective tissue are derived from neural crest.

25) a. Distant object fixation usually worsens the nystagmus. On the other hand, purposely induced esotropia or near fixation is used to suppress the nystagmus (nystagmus blocking syndrome). The pursuit movement in a normal person is towards the direction of the optokinetic drum, and quick phases in the opposite direction. In congenital nystagmus, the reversed is observed.

26) c. In England and Wales, treatment can be provided in the young person's best interests without parental consent, although the views of parents may be important in assessing his best interests. At the age of 16, he can be presumed to have the capacity to consent. Under 16, he may have the capacity to consent, depending on his maturity and ability to understand what is involved. He may have the capacity to consent to a straightforward, relatively risk-free treatment, however not necessarily to complex treatments involving high risks or serious consequences.

27) c. Only the upper eyelids are involved. It can be unilateral or bilateral. Patients experience bouts of painless lid oedema for several days. The recurrence results in stretching of the skin with eventual atrophy of the lid tissue. Patients can present with blepharoptosis, thinning of the lid skin, conjunctival chemosis and injection.

28) a. The mean deviation refers to the average deviation of sensitivity at each test location from age-adjusted normal population values, which provides an indication of the degree of generalised loss in the field. The pattern standard deviation represents a summary measurement of the average deviation of individual visual field sensitivity values from the normal 'hill of vision' after correcting for any overall sensitivity differences. The corrected pattern standard deviation is the pattern standard deviation after taking into consideration the short-

term fluctuation (an indication of consistency of response assessed by testing ten pre-selected points twice and analysing the difference).

29) b. Relative risk = $\dfrac{\text{Disease incidence in exposed group}}{\text{Disease incidence in non-exposed group}}$

Attributable risk = Disease incidence in exposed group – disease incidence in non-exposed group

Odd ratio = $\dfrac{\text{Odds of subject with disease exposed to risk factor}}{\text{Odds that subject without disease exposed to risk factor}}$

30) b. Irregular astigmatism is usually corneal in nature. It can also cause by the different refractive indices in a cataractous lens however this is more uncommon.

31) b. The normalised colour scales are not fixed and tend to vary from patient to patient; therefore it's pertinent to pay attention to the actual numerical scale rather than just the colour changes.

32) c. Venous changes are seen in diabetic retinopathy. Hypertensive retinopathy only affects the retinal arteries. The venous defects seen are at the arteriovenous junction and secondary to arterial effect. Hypertensive retinopathy can cause choroidopathy. Elschnig spots (grey-black spots surrounded by yellow ring indicative of focal choroidal and RPE infarct) and Siegrist streaks (yellow linear flecks and pigmentation along choroidal vessels indicative of arterial fibrinoid necrosis) are secondary to this condition.

33) a. The Jarisch–Herxheimer reaction is due to release of TNF-α, IL-6 and IL-8. It is seen in half of patients with primary syphilis and up to 90% of patients with secondary syphilis on IV penicillin treatment. It occurs about 8 hours after the first injection and usually consists of mild fever, malaise and headache lasting several hours. In neurosyphilis, the reaction, although more uncommon, may be severe and exacerbate the clinical manifestations. Prednisolone given for 24 hours prior to therapy may ameliorate the reaction but there is little evidence to support its use. Penicillin should not be withheld because of the Jarisch–Herxheimer reaction; since it is not a dose-related phenomenon, there is no value in giving a smaller dose.

34) c. The involved pupil usually does not react or reacts poorly and irregularly to light stimulation but constrict on adduction or downgaze. The pupil will appear to constrict more during convergence than to light (pseudo-Argyll Robertson). This is possibly due to the innervations of the pupillary sphincter muscle by the medial or inferior rectus fibres.

35) d. The 30Hz flicker stimulus is performed with a rod-saturating background illumination. The rods have a poor temporal resolution and are unable to respond to a stimulus presented at this rate. This is a pure cone test, and cone dysfunction will produce an abnormal result. The b-wave reflects the activity of Muller cells. It is maximal with a bright light stimulus in a scotopic condition.

36) d.

37) c. An acute inflammation is initiated by a vascular phase. Histamine, kinins and prostaglandins increase the blood vessels' permeability and calibre. Unlike an immune response an acute inflammation is neither adaptive, specific nor exhibit memory.

38) a. Stereopsis can be detected but not measured by synoptophore. The synoptophore can also evaluate the potential binocular function in the presence of a manifest squint. It can also detect suppression.

39) b. The risk factors include POAG, pigmentary glaucoma, family history of glaucoma, high myopes, and diabetics.

40) a. Before entering the orbit, the sympathetic fibres travel on the surface of ophthalmic artery. As it emerges into the orbit, it joins the nasociliary nerve which form one of the divisions of the long ciliary nerve, and it innervates the ciliary ganglion then continue as short ciliary nerve to reach the ciliary body and pupil dilator.

41) c. Creatinine kinase is increased in myocyte death in cardiac disease. Sarcoidosis can infiltrate the heart albeit this is rare. The main symptoms are ventricular dysrhythmias and conduction defect.

42) b. Stromal disease is secondary to a hypersensitivity reaction to the herpes virus antigen. The trigeminal ganglion is the sole reservoir of herpes simplex during latency. Once the person is infected, cell-mediated immunity develops. In some individuals this response is poor and recurrent attacks occur. Immunosuppression can also cause recrudescence of HSV. The virus can also auto-inoculate into sites of trauma and present as painful blisters/pustules which may be seen for example on the fingers of healthcare workers ('herpetic whitlow').

43) d. Not all lasers are polarised. However, all would be coherent, monochromatic and collimated. Coherence means the light rays are phase-synchronized. Monochromaticity implies light rays of the same frequency. Collimated refers to same direction of travel.

44) a. The disease can only manifest in a male, and cannot be transmitted to his sons. However, all his daughters will be carriers. Half of the daughter's sons will have the disease and 50% of daughters carriers.

45) b. The peaks occur when there is a large change in the refractive indices. The peaks occur at the cornea anterior and posterior surfaces, lens anterior and posterior surfaces and the ILM.

46) c. Pilocarpine is a direct-acting parasympathomimetic. It decreases accommodative effort and can be used to treat esotropia secondary to excessive accommodation. Although it reverses a phenylephrine mydriasis, it will not do the same for atropine.

47) a. The listed conditions affect some part of the connective tissues in the vitreous or retinal except pseudoxanthoma elasticum. The latter affects the elastin in the Bruch layer.

48) d. Spindle cells are found in choroidal melanoma. Embryonal calls are the most common type of rhabdomyosarcoma; alveolar has the worse and pleomorphic the best prognoses.

49) d. Apart from an accurate history of the event, a detailed description of the ocular and systemic examination findings with drawings should be recorded. Photographic documentation of the extent of the injuries is helpful and should always be considered. An objective documentation may be useful in supporting claims filed with solicitors and insurance companies. In a road traffic accident, it is recommended to note down the names of the driver, first aid provider and eyewitnesses. A statement from the latter should also be sort if he/she is present during the clinical consultation with the patient.

50) b. Tears contains (in order of frequency) IgA, IgG, IgM; lactoferrin (free radical scavenger), lysozyme and betalysin.

51) b. The Royal College recommends that if the local rates of endophthalmitis over a properly audited time frame are similar to those reported in the Bolton study (0.055%), continuation with the current preventative measures are in place is reasonable. However, if local rates are higher, then intracameral cefuroxime may be added as part of a package of measures to lower the rate of endophthalmitis after a suitable analysis of processes has taken place.

52) c. The Mantoux test is negative up to 50% of patients with severe tuberculosis. In the majority of patients first infected with tuberculosis (primary tuberculosis), no or vague symptoms are present. Respiratory symptoms usually manifest 1- 2 months later.

53) d. The aim of economic evaluation is to ensure that the benefits from health care programs implemented are greater than the opportunity cost of such programs by addressing questions of allocative efficiency, technical efficiency, cost and consequences (effectiveness and benefits).

54) a. Sun-flower cataracts present in patients with Wilson disease; stellate posterior subcapsular cataract in myotonic dystrophy and posterior cortical cataract in neurofibromatosis type 2.

55) a. MRI diffuse-weighted image scan provides more sensitive visualisation of an acute infarct than FLAIR / T2 weighted scan. A CT scans is better for acute haemorrhage. CTA and MRA are indicated in aneurysm, carotid disease and carotid cavernous fistula.

56) c. Hemifacial spasm is usually caused by compression of the facial nerve root at the cerebellopontine angle by a blood vessel (or tumour). Facial myokymia signifies a dysfunction at the seventh nerve nucleus or fascicle in the pons.

57) d. The failure rate is about 50-65% is 5 years. The effectiveness decreases with time. Elderly patients usually have good IOP reduction with laser trabeculoplasty. The procedure can be repeated however, the success rate is less.

58) b. In a normal person, about half (or just slightly more) of the optic nerve fibres cross at the optic chiasm. In albinism, this can be up to 90%, causing neural disorganisation at the lateral geniculate body. Patients usually have <6/60 vision due to foveal hypoplasia. They are likely to have squints, nystagmus and high refractive errors. Oculocutaneous albinism is an autosomal recessive condition.

59) c. Chloroquine causes retinotoxicity.

60) d. Peripheral ulcerative keratitis is caused by autoimmune diseases and not herpes zoster infection. Autoimmune complex are deposited at the end arteries near the limbus resulting in an ischaemic event and release of metalloproteinases.

61) c. The smaller chart represents the paretic muscle eye and the larger chart the overacting eye. The former reveals the maximum restriction in the direction of action of the affected muscle. The larger chart shows the maximum expansion in the direction of action of the yoke muscle. Each square represents 10PD and gives a good estimate of the angle of deviation. With the passage of time, the secondary contracture of the ipsilateral antagonist muscle will show up as an overaction. The result of this is secondary inhibitional palsy of the antagonist of the yoke muscle which shows up as an underaction. Eventually the two charts become more similar.

62) a. Increased glycosaminoglycans are secreted by inflammatory cells in the extraocular muscles in thyroid orbitopathy. This causes an osmotic change in the muscle and oedema ensues secondary to water imbibition.

63) b. Patients are usually born with non-progressive ophthalmoplegia. The aetiology is due to abnormal development of oculomotor subnuclei resulting in anomalous innervations of the extraocular musculature. The eyes are usually frozen in downgaze and abduction, with very little or no ability to adduct, depress or elevate.

64) d. Vigabatrin is an anti-epileptic drug. Peripheral visual filed loss is an early side-effect and patients are usually asymptomatic at this stage. Patients taking vigabatrin should undergo a visual field test 6 monthly for the first 5 years followed by annual test. The perimetry should be at least 45 degrees of eccentricity. If a defect is detected, perimetry should be repeated within 1 month before considering cessation of vigabatrin. If the drug is discontinued, perimetry should be performed at a future date to monitor the field loss.

65) c. Toxoplasmosis retinitis usually presents when the CD4+ count is less than 200/μl. The conditions that occur when the CD4+ count is 200 - 500/μl includes herpes zoster, herpes simplex, tuberculosis retinitis, aspergillosis and molluscum contagiosum.

66) b. This is type 1 error. Type 2 error is 'c'.

67) a. The near-infrared wavelength of ICG can penetrate the RPE, choroid and overlying haemorrhage. It is helpful in occult or poorly defined CNV and to detect any leakage in a fibrovascular pigment epithelial detachment.

68) c. The other drugs that can cause optic neuropathy include vigabatrin, amiodarone, hydroxyquinolone, penicillamine, cisplatin and vincristine.

69) d. Recurrence tends to be more difficult to treat due to deeper tissue invasion and more likely differentiation into the sclerosing subtype.

70) a. Retinoblastoma cells derive from neuroepithelial cells and have the potential to differentiate into photoreceptors or Muller cells. In order of increasing maturity Homer-Wright rosettes, neuroblasts, Flexner-Wintersteiner rosettes, early retinal cells, fleurettes, immature photoreceptors cells. Unlike choroidal melanoma, the type of cells is not a prognosticator.

71) b. There is absence of intraocular inflammation in PIC. APMPPE and serpiginous choroidopathy cause mild vitritis. Birdshot retinochoroidopathy causes moderate vitritis which may lead to cystoid macular oedema.

72) a. Treating paired measurements as unpaired samples will artificially increase the sample size and lead to inaccurate analyses. The assumptions for a paired t-test are the outcome variable has a

continuous scale and the differences between the samples follows a Gaussian distribution.

73) c. The calcium-channel antibodies are present in Lambert-Eaton syndrome. This is a paraneoplastic syndrome commonly related to small-cell bronchial carcinoma. The condition causes defective acetylcholine release at the neuromuscular junction. Antibodies to acetylcholine receptor are deposited at the postsynaptic membranes, causing interference with and later destruction of the acetylcholine receptors. Antibodies against muscle-specific receptor tyrosine kinase have been identified in anti-AChR antibody negative cases. Thymic hyperplasia is found in 70% of myasthenia gravis patients below the age of 40. In about 10%, a thymic tumour is found (the incidence increasing with age) antibodies to striated muscle can be demonstrated in some of these patients.

74) d. Miller Fisher syndrome is a variant of Guillain-Barre syndrome. A triad of areflexia, ophthalmoplegia and ataxia occur. Unlike the latter, it does not cause acute motor axonal neuropathy. The majority of patients have GQ1b IgG autoantibodies in their serum. Recovery occurs with time and is usually complete. The serology also improves with clinical improvement.

75) b. Endothelial graft rejection occurs in 20-30% of grafts over a 5 year period in the UK. The failure rate is 25-35% over the same period. Some 5-10% of graft rejections result in failure. The majority of the rejection episodes occur between 3-18 months post-PK in the UK.

76) b. A traumatic retinal dialysis is usually repaired with a scleral buckle. Heavy tamponade is usually indicated for complicated vitreoretinal surgery which includes penetrating injury detachment, multiple retinal tear inferiorly, posterior break detachment, choroidal detachment, and severe tractional detachment.

77) c. Tetracaine has the longer lasting analgesic effect, although it causes more stinging. Benoxinate is bacteriostatic against staphylococcus and pseudomonas, therefore proxymethocaine is the preferable anaesthetic for corneal scrape. Oxybuprocaine and tetracaine are toxic and should not be used systemically.

78) b. These individuals have no symptoms unless extreme circumstances cause anoxia. Sickle cell trait gives some protection against *Plasmodium falciparum* malaria and consequently the sickle gene has been seen as an example of a balanced polymorphism. The blood count and film of a sickle cell trait patient are normal. The diagnosis is made by a positive sickle test or by Hb electrophoresis. Sickle-cell C and sickle-cell thalassaemia diseases have the worse retinopathy.

79) a. Histologically, an acquired melanocytic naevus pigmented can show naevus cells at the epidermal and dermal junction (known as junctional naevus); in both epidermis and dermis (compound naevus); or mainly in the dermis layer (intradermal naevus). Melanoma cells are usually found in the epidermis layer in a lid melanoma. A Kaposi sarcoma shows proliferation of spindle cells, vessels and mitosis within the dermis layer.

80) c. The amplitude (not the latency) of pattern VEP can be employed as an objective measure of the visual acuity. When the checked pattern size is reduced to the degree where it cannot be resolved by the eye, the cortical response subsides. At a check size of 15 min arc, visual acuity of at least 6/18 is required for a cortical response. In acute demyelination of the optic nerve, the VEP is usually undetectable. When the visual acuity has improved, the VEP tends to show almost normal amplitudes but remains permanently delayed by at least 30ms.

81) d. The distribution of χ^2 is a skew deviation. Chi-square serves as a measure of how different the observed frequencies are from the expected frequencies. A large value of χ^2 indicates a lack of agreement, while a small one indicates close agreement between what was expected in the null hypothesis and what actually occurred.

82) b. Pleomorphic lacrimal gland adenomas and meningiomas have a tendency to displace their surrounding tissues. Malignant tumours tend to cause destruction by invading the tissue in their vicinity. Cancerous cells display a higher nuclear to cytoplasmic ratio. The rate and frequency of mitoses are high.

83) c. Only a cerebellopontine angle lesion causes the combination of V^1, VI (distant diplopia), VII, and VIII palsies. Gradenigo syndrome is due to extradural abscess at the petrous apex following complicated otitis media. It affects the V, VI, VII and VIII nerves, however, causes facial pain in the distribution of V nerve. Ramsay Hunt syndrome involves the V^1 and VII nerves.

84) a. Silicone oil can cause various complications. Early glaucoma occurs due to pupillary block and this can be prevented by an inferior (Ando) iridectomy. Late glaucoma is due to emulsified oil blocking the trabecular meshwork. Cataract, filamentary keratitis, ERM and band keratopathy are not uncommon. Emulsified oil can results in anterior uveitis, subconjunctival and subretinal cyst formation.

85) d. An evisceration is preferred for refractory panophthalmitis. Cutting the optic nerve (in enucleation) results in exposing the meninges. There is a higher risk of meningitis for an infected eye.

86) c. Filamentary keratitis usually results from dysfunctional aqueous and mucus productions. Loose epithelium strands occur and abnormal thick mucus anchors to these. Blinking causes the eyelid to rub against the mobile mucus, hence stimulating the sensitive corneal nerve. Filamentary keratitis can be due to keratoconjunctivitis sicca, epithelial instability (recurrent corneal erosion, refractive surgery), neurotrophic keratitis (herpes simplex and zoster) and prolonged eye patching and blepharospasm.

87) b. Gradual systemic corticosteroids withdrawal must be considered on an individual basis. Factors including the likelihood of disease relapse, adrenal suppression and duration of corticosteroid treatment must be taken into account. Gradual withdrawal should be considered for those who have received more than 40mg daily in the morning for more than a week, repeated evening doses, received more than 3 weeks of treatment, taken a short course but within a year of stopping long-term steroid therapy, or receiving another repeated course of at least 3 weeks after stopping multiple short courses recently.

88) c. Malingers usually can fake a Humphrey perimetry even in the presence of reliable indices. Goldmann perimetry can reveal spiraling or crossing isopters. Frisby test requires both eyes to resolve a disparity measured (600 to 15 seconds of arc) to see the image in the plates. The red-green duochrome induces a patient to read with an eye that supposedly cannot see by making the patient think that he is using both eyes. The eye behind the red lens will see letters on both sides of the chart, while the green lens eye will see only those letters on the green side.

89) a. Antithrombin deficiency is a cause of venous thromboembolism. Antiphospholipid syndrome, protein S and protein C deficiencies cause arterial and venous thromboembolism.

90) All patients who enter a clinical trial should be followed up, even if they abandon the treatment protocol, since exclusion of these patients can introduce bias. Patient data are required to be eliminated safely after a trial has been completed to protect patient confidentiality. When a clinical trial is in progress, it is ethically necessary, to analyse the interim accrued data. If one treatment is found to be superior, it may be necessary to stop the trial so that all subjects may receive the best treatment. However, a clinical trial should not be stopped as soon as a significant result at the 5% level has been achieved since this does not take into consideration the effect of repeated statistical testing. The advice of a statistician should be sort.

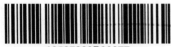

Printed in Great Britain
by Amazon.co.uk, Ltd.,
Marston Gate.